Essential Skills

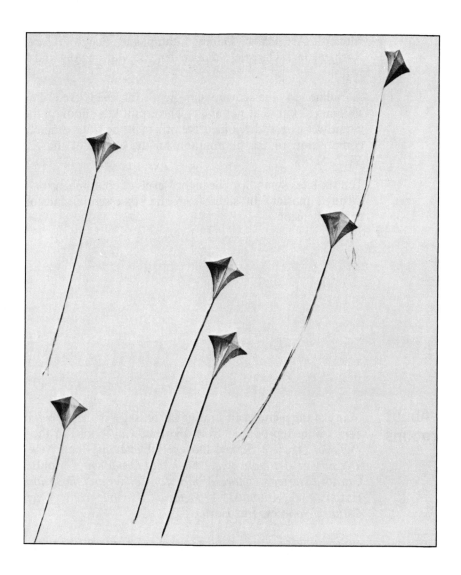

Revised Edition

About the Cover

The breeze was fresh this bright day in May, and gaily-colored kites appeared like spring swallows, darting across the blue sky over Rhode Island's Narragansett Bay. Photographer Tony Botelho was there to capture on film the kite-flights of Christy Menard, Art Pelosi, Danny Champagne, Peggy Hulsey, John Rathjen, Jack Christie, Stephen Jencks, Marion Alig and Megen Mills.

A salute to the rowboaters who retrieved the "diamond-spinnaker" kite that got away! The errant kite shook in the wind like a wet dog and rejoined the others in the sky, completing the composition of the photograph on the covers of the *Essential Skills Series*.

The six kites symbolize the higher levels of comprehension gained through mastery of skills from the six essential categories of comprehension.

About the Illustrations

Many of the pictures illustrating the passages in the *Essential Skills Series* were reproduced from the following books in the *Dover Pictorial Archive Series*, Dover Publications, Inc., New York: *Treasury of Art Nouveau, Design and Ornament*, Carol Belanger Grafton; *Harter's Picture Archive for Collage and Illustration*, Jim Harter; and *Animals: A Pictorial Archive from Nineteenth-Century Sources*, Jim Harter.

Other illustrations are by Christine Orciuch, Deborah Christie, Howard Lewis and Thomas Ewing Malloy.

Essential Skills Series

Essential Skills Book 2

Walter Pauk, Ph.D.
Director, Reading Research Center
Cornell University

Revised Edition

Jamestown Publishers
Providence, Rhode Island

Essential Skills Series
No. 302, Book 2

Cover Design by Deborah Hulsey Christie, adapted from the Original Design by Stephen R. Anthony

Text Design by Deborah Hulsey Christie

Printed in the United States AL

88 89 90 91 92 11 10 9 8 7

ISBN 0-89061-221-8

Preface

Practice Makes Perfect

Why do some students shoot baskets over and over again and others skate and reskate the same routine? These beginners know that practice makes perfect. Not only do beginners know this, but pros do too. For what other reason do they work at baseball and football week after week before the opening dates?

Value of Practice

The pros know the value of practice, but they also know the value of something else. They know that practice without *instruction* and *guidance* does not automatically lead to improvement. That's why they have the best coaches that money can buy.

And so it is with developing the skills of reading. There must be the right kind of practicing and the right kind of coaching.

First, a word about practice. In this book the right kind of practice is provided by twenty-five highly interesting and carefully selected passages. Here is material enough on which to grow and keep growing.

Value of Coaching

Now about coaching! Good coaching takes the form of instruction and guidance. In this book the instruction is straightforward and uncomplicated. It puts you directly on the right track, and better still, you are kept on the right track by two unusual systems of guidance. The first system is the uniquely designed, six-way question format which makes sure that every ounce of practice is directed toward improvement. Nothing is wasted!

Diagnostic Chart

The second system of guidance is the Diagnostic Chart. This chart is no ordinary gimmick. In truth, it provides the most dignified form of diagnosis and guidance yet devised. It provides instantaneous and continuous diagnosis and gentle but certain self-guidance. It yields information directly to the student. This form of self-guidance leads to the goal of all education: the goal of self-teaching.

Acknowledgments Now, I want to make some acknowledgments, especially to the students who were the guinea pigs. Afterwards I told them so, but they said, "We didn't mind even then. And now that it is over, we're all the happier because we know how much we've learned." But what the students did not know was how much I learned from them. For this I thank them all, class after class.

I direct especial thanks to Linda Browning, Anita DuBose, and Karen Duddy for handling the almost countless number of selections, writing and refining the questions and making sure that the series kept moving: all, a most demanding task.

Finally, I am most grateful to authors, editors and publishers who have generously given permission to quote and reprint in this book from works written and published by them. The books quoted in the text and used as sources of reading extracts are listed in the back of the book.

Walter Pauk

Contents

To the Instructor

Selection of Passages

All of us believe in this truism: to learn to read, a person must read. But, placing a book in front of a student won't automatically promote reading.

This last sentence brings up another truism: you can lead a horse to water, but you can't make it drink. To tempt a horse, the water must be clear, cool and clean.

To tempt the student, the passages must be genuinely fascinating. Knowing this, we packed each book with twenty-five "I can't put the book down" type of passages.

Each passage had to meet at least the following criteria: *high interest level, appropriate readability level* and *factual accuracy of contents.* High interest was assured by choosing passages from popular magazines that appeal to a wide range of readers. The readability level of each passage was assessed by applying Dr. Edward B. Fry's *Formula for Estimating Readability,* thus enabling the arrangement of passages on a single grade level within each book. The factual accuracy of the passages is high because they were written by professional writers whose works are recognized and respected.

The Great Value of Questions

Dr. Mortimer J. Adler says that the overall secret for improving one's reading can be boiled down to knowing how to keep awake while reading. He means more than keeping one's eyes open. He means keeping one's mind open and active.

One sure-fire way to do this is to keep trying to answer questions while reading. Questions not only keep one's mind awake, but also keep the mind active, not letting it get flabby. Here's a good story that makes the same point.

> To keep their fish alive for the fresh-fish markets, the owners of fishing boats used a water-filled floating tank. The fish remained alive all right, but they were never firm, always flabby. One captain, however, always brought back firm, fresh, active fish. His fish always received a higher price.

One day he revealed his secret: "You see," he said, "for every hundred herrings I put into my tank, I put in one catfish. It is true that the catfish eat five or six of the herrings on the trip back to port, but the catfish keep the rest alert and constantly active. That's why my herring arrive in beautiful condition."

The work of the catfish, in this book, is done by the six essential questions (subject matter, supporting details, conclusion, clarifying devices, vocabulary in context, and main idea). These questions keep the minds of students alert, active and in beautiful condition.

The main idea questions in this book are not the usual multiple-choice variety. Given four statements, the students are asked to recognize the main idea of the passage. They also tell why each of the other three does not express the main idea; the students identify one statement as too narrow, one as too broad and one as merely a detail.

By asking these six types of questions in each passage, students quickly learn to read with a questioning and anticipating attitude. This attitude, necessary for high comprehension, is easily transferred to other material such as the textbook.

The Diagnostic Chart

Those who used the first edition of these books had high praise for the Diagnostic Chart. In sum, this is what they said.

The Diagnostic Chart is truly ingenious because it is, in fact, a self-diagnosing instrument. The Chart instantly, simply and continually shows students their strengths and weaknesses.

Here is how the Chart works. The six questions for each passage are always in the same order. For example, the question designed to teach the skill of making *conclusions* is always in the number three position, and the question designed to teach the skill of identifying *clarifying devices* is always in the number four position, and so forth. This innovation of keeping the questions in order sets the stage for the smooth functioning of the Chart.

The Chart works automatically when the letters of the answers are placed in the spaces on the Chart. Even after completing one passage, the Chart will reveal the type or types of questions answered correctly as well as the types answered incorrectly. But more important, the Chart will identify the types of questions missed consistently. More persuasive identification is possible after three or more passages have been completed. By then, a pattern can be observed. For example, if the answers to question number three (making conclusions) are incorrect for all three passages, or on three out of four, then this weakness shows up automatically.

Once a weakness is revealed, instruct the students to take the following steps: First, turn back to the instructional pages to study the section in which the topic is discussed. Second, go back to read again the questions in that particular category that were missed; then, with the correct answers in mind, read the entire passage again, trying to see how the author developed the answers to the questions. Third, on succeeding passages, put forth extra effort to answer correctly the questions in that particular category. Fourth, if the difficulty still persists, arrange for a conference with the instructor.

To the Student

How do readers get the meaning from written words? To get meaning, readers need to know at least six essential skills.

1. Subject Matter — Readers need to know how to concentrate or focus on the writing. This helps them learn what the writing is about.
2. Main Idea — Readers need to know how to grasp the main idea or point of the writing.
3. Supporting Details — Readers need to be able to connect supporting details to the ideas.
4. Conclusions — Readers should be able to come to conclusions or guess endings based on the ideas.
5. Clarifying Devices — Readers should be able to note the writer's methods of making the points clear and alive.
6. Vocabulary in Context — Readers must know what the words in the writing mean.

Let's take a closer look at these six skills.

**Concentration/
Subject Matter**

One thing readers often say is, "I can't concentrate!" But there is a sure, fast cure. There is no better way to gain concentration when reading than this. Read the first few lines. Then ask yourself these questions: "What is this passage about?" "What is the subject matter?"

If you don't ask these questions, here's what may happen. Your eyes will move across the lines of print. Yet your mind will be thinking of other things.

But if you ask the questions, you will most likely get an answer, thus achieving concentration. Let's see if this method works. Here are the first lines of a passage:

> Wood ducks are the most beautiful ducks in North America. Once they were rare. Now — if you have sharp eyes and can keep quiet — you might see them in almost any woodland along streams and ponds.

After reading this, you can see that the author will talk about the wood duck. Now that your mind is on the trail, the chances are good it will follow the author's idea line by line. Thus, you will *concentrate* on the building of the subject matter.

Let's try the method again. Here are a few lines from another passage:

> Of all the little animals in the world, the Columbian ground squirrel is one of the liveliest and friendliest. It is nicknamed "picket pin." This is because it sits as stiff and straight as a stake in the ground.

Again, you most likely had no trouble picking out the subject. It is the Columbian ground squirrel.

Main Idea

Once the subject matter has been grasped, it is time for the next question. Ask yourself, "What is the author's main idea?" "What point is the passage trying to make?"

With such questions in mind, you can be sure an answer will often pop up. But when no questions are asked, all things seem the same. Nothing stands out. The reader will not see the point of the passage.

Let's look at another passage. This time we will find the main idea.

> Wood ducks never nest on the ground as most ducks do, but in a big hole in a tree. Trees with big holes in them are hard to find.

You don't have the full passage to read, so I will tell you the answer. The main point is that with fewer and fewer old, dead trees with big holes in them, we will have fewer and fewer wood ducks.

Thus, when questions are asked, the reader is acting upon the content. Reading becomes a two-way street with both reader and writer engaged. In a sense, the reader talks with the author. So the passage comes to life. Reading then is a joy.

Supporting Details Do we like details? Of course we do. In long pieces of writing, main ideas are like the bones. They are the skeleton of the writing. The details are the flesh. They give the writing fullness and life.

Details are used to support the main ideas. So the term *supporting details* fits well. These supporting details come in many forms. The most common forms are examples, definitions, comparisons, contrasts, repetitions and descriptions.

The author of "The Wood Duck" lets us know that the passage is about wood ducks. Next, the author makes sure we learn that the point is that without trees with holes, the wood duck will not nest. Thus, there would be fewer wood ducks.

Now that we are involved in this problem, the author gives us details on how we can provide trees with holes in them. The author *describes* how we can build a wood duck nesting box. Here's the excerpt:

> Why don't you and your parents put up a wood duck nesting box right now? It would be about two feet (about .61 meters) high and ten inches (about 25.4 centimeters) square. Make the entry hole about four inches (about 10.2 centimeters) across. Use rough lumber on the inside, so the ducklings can climb up the sides to the hole. Put wood shavings on the bottom. In these the duck will lay her eggs. To keep her eggs warm, she covers them with her own feathers. If you can't find a tree near the water, you will need a post. Place the box ten to thirty feet (about 3.1 to 9.1 meters) high.

You can see in the above passage how important details are in telling a story. Details let the reader see what's going on. They paint a vivid picture of the action. They may tell how to do something. They may tell how something happened.

In long passages there will also be sub-ideas. It is important to be careful not to mistake a sub-idea for a main idea. Sub-ideas are broader than details. But sub-ideas are still not the main point. The main idea has to do with the whole passage. The sub-idea has to do with just part of it. Note that in the next sample, the sub-idea is about the food that wood ducks eat. The whole passage is not about food. Thus, food is *not* the main idea. For the most part, you will see that a sub-idea takes the space of one paragraph. Often, the topic sentence of the paragraph is a statement of a sub-idea.

The following excerpts show how the author groups and structures supporting details around the sub-ideas that are stated in topic sentences. A sub-idea will hold a group of details together.

> Wood ducks eat acorns and all kinds of nuts. Their stomachs (or gizzards) have strong muscles. They can break the hardest nuts, some that you could barely crack with a hammer, in their stomachs. Wood ducks like berries, duckweed and insects. But best of all they like to eat spiders. That's ice cream to them.

The topic sentence is the first sentence. It states that the sub-idea is the foods wood ducks eat. Next, the author describes how the newly hatched ducklings get down to the ground from the nest.

Here are more details grouped around a sub-idea.

> Sometimes they nest in holes up in trees that are twice as high as a flagpole. Just think, the baby ducklings must jump to the ground the day they hatch. They don't get hurt, though, because they're light, like little puffs of cotton. The mother stands at the foot of the tree and calls and calls. The ducklings peek out of the hole. Then, like little paratroopers, they jump quickly, one right after the other, to join their mother. She must then hurry them to the pond where they're safe.

Thus, one of the main jobs of *supporting details* is to give some fullness to the passage. The passage would be just a boring, skimpy statement of the main idea with its bare-boned sub-ideas if not for details. The details give the passage life.

Conclusion   The reader will move through a passage, grasping the main and sub-ideas and their details. It is then common for the reader to start to guess a conclusion or ending to the story. Such guesses are part of the sport of reading. Often, the author gives the reader an ending. In such a case, the joy of reading lies in the fact that the reader finds out the guess was right. But the ending may not be given. The reader then will try to guess the ending that is hinted by the author.

The conclusion from the excerpts just read about the wood duck is in having the reader see the pleasure of observing a wood duck. The final sentence is this:

> If you're lucky, though, and if your (duck) house is in place before the ice melts, you will have a wood duck family in the summer.

In a passage called "From Pond to Prairie," the author has this conclusion:

> Finally, there is no longer much open water. The pond has disappeared. Depending on the kinds of plants that have filled it, the pond may be called a bog or a marsh. As changes continue for many more years, the bog may become a forest.

The skillful reader is like a detective. This reader follows the story, always thinking, "Where is the author leading me?" "What's the final point?" "What's the conclusion?" And the reader, like a detective, must try to guess the conclusion, changing the guess if necessary as the story unfolds.

Clarifying Devices   The author uses clarifying devices to make the points in the story clear and alive. In a sense, the *topic sentence* may be thought of as a clarifying device. It is often placed at the start of a paragraph. In this way, the author gives the reader a quick point of focus.

The point of the passage becomes clear after reading it.

But more often, by clarifying devices, we mean the literary devices in the passage. These are words or phrases which keep the ideas, sub-ideas and details in clear focus and in order.

Authors use literary devices to make details clear and interesting. An example of a device is the *metaphor,* as in "But best of all they like to eat spiders. *That's ice cream to them.*"

One more literary device is the *simile. "Like little paratroopers,* they (the ducklings) jump quickly, one right after the other, to join their mother," is a simile. The simile helps the reader imagine a vivid scene. It brings to the mind of the reader something known — paratroopers. Then it compares the known idea to the ducklings' jump from their nest to make a fresh, new idea. It is fun to imagine the little ducks copying real paratroopers jumping from a plane.

Besides metaphors and similes, other *clarifying devices* are organizational patterns. One common pattern is to unfold the events in the order of time. Thus, one thing happens first and then another and another, and so forth.

The time pattern orders the event. The event may take place in the span of five minutes. It may last hundreds of years. A time pattern may be used to relate the habits of an animal from its birth to its death.

You should learn to find these literary devices. They help you to understand the passage and speed your reading.

Vocabulary in Context

A reader who does not know what the author's words mean may not understand the passage. A reader should look up in the dictionary the unknown words.

Also a reader may understand only the general meaning of the word. But sometimes a more *exact* meaning is needed to grasp the passage fully. A reader who places a general meaning on a word may end up with a blurred picture of the idea. An exact meaning will give the reader a full and clear picture.

For instance, in the next excerpt are two common words that many people feel they already know. Thus, they don't see the need to look them up in the dictionary. But few people know the exact meaning of these words.

> Depending on the kinds of plants that have filled it, the pond may be called a *bog* or a *marsh.*

Do you know the difference between a bog and a marsh? Is there a difference? If so, what is it? How would your mental picture change if you knew?

Looking up words for their exact meanings is rewarding. A precise vocabulary leads to true understanding.

You may find it troublesome to look up words you feel you already know. But you should get into this habit to improve your reading. Of course, words you do not know must always be looked up. You would most likely need a dictionary for these words:

> Nothing could appear more *benign* than a field aglow with daisies, goldenrod and Queen Anne's lace.

> *Sphinxlike,* it crouches among the flowers until the desired insect wanders within reach.

The dictionary is like a stock market. Here you exchange fuzzy meanings for exact meanings. You get new meanings for unknown words. All this is at no cost. It takes just a flip of your finger.

Answering the Main Idea Question

To be able to find the main idea of the things you read is important. It is one of the best reading skills you can learn. The main idea questions in this book are not the ones you've seen where you pick just the right answer. Instead, each main idea question is made up of four statements. Two of the statements refer to just parts of the passage. One of these is a *detail.* It states a point. But that point has little to do with the passage as a whole. The next statement is *too narrow.* It tells more than the detail statement. Still, it's too specific to tell about the main point of the passage. The "too narrow" statement is often a sub-idea.

The last two statements deal with the whole passage. One is *too broad.* It is too general and too vague to be a good main idea statement. The final statement is the *main idea.* It tells *who* or *what* the point of the passage is. The main idea statement answers the question *does what?* or *is what?* also.

Read the sample passage below. Then follow the instructions in the box. The answer to each part of the main idea question has been filled in for you. The score for each answer has also been marked.

Sample

The steel trap's jaws had caught the coyote midway across the foot. The pain must have been awful. Yet the coyote never stopped trying to tear loose. It had dug a circle about six inches (about 15.2 centimeters) deep, stretching the full length of the steel chain.

Two young boys out hiking saw this trapped coyote. They hurried to a nearby ranch. The ranch owner heard them out and came to help.

They held the coyote's neck down firmly with hoe handles. Then they opened the trap's jaws. The coyote slipped free. But the animal stayed there, just looking at its helpers. Perhaps it was wondering what makes some people demons and others saints.

The animal had to be gently nudged before it would leave. At last, it hobbled off a short distance. Then it turned, pausing to look again at the good people who had spared its life.

	Answer	Score
Mark the main idea	M	(10)
Mark the statement that is a detail	D	5
Mark the statement that is too narrow	N	5
Mark the statement that is too broad	B	5

a. Two young boys helped to free a trapped coyote.
   [This statement is one that gathers all the important points. It gives a correct picture of the main idea in a brief way: (1) two young boys, (2) a trapped coyote, and (3) freeing it.]

   M (10)

b. Kind hearts set free a doomed coyote.
   [This statement is too broad. It doesn't state *who* set the coyote free. It doesn't tell *why* it was doomed.]

   B (5)

c. Hoe handles were used to hold the coyote down.
   [This is just one of many details found in the passage. It has little to do with the passage as a whole.]

   D (5)

d. A steel trap was opened to set a coyote free.
   [Opening the trap is *part* of the main idea. But any main idea statement must give the chief actors credit. It must mention the two boys who set the coyote free.]

   N (5)

Getting the Most Out of This Book   The following steps could be called "tricks of the trade." Your teachers might call them "rules for learning." It doesn't matter what they are called. What does matter is that they work.

Think About the Title

A famous language expert told me a "trick" to use when I read. "The first thing to do is to read the title. Then spend a few moments thinking about it."

Writers spend much time thinking up good titles. They try to pack a lot of meaning into them. It makes sense, then, for you to spend a few seconds trying to dig out some meaning. These few moments of thought will give you a head start on a passage.

Thinking about the title can help you in another way, too. It helps you concentrate on a passage before you begin reading. Why does this happen? Thinking about the title fills your head full of thoughts about the passage. There's no room for anything else to get in to break concentration.

The Dot System

Here is a method that will speed up your reading. It also builds comprehension at the same time.

Spend a few moments with the title. Then read *quickly* through the passage. Next, without looking back, answer the six questions by placing a dot in the box next to each answer of your choice. The dots will be your "unofficial" answers. For the main idea question (question six), place your dot in the box next to the statement that you think is the main idea.

The dot system helps by making you think hard on your first, *fast* reading. The practice you gain by trying to grasp and remember ideas makes you a stronger reader.

The Check-Mark System

You have now answered all of the questions with a dot. Next, read the passage once more *carefully*. This time, make your final answer to each question with a check mark (✓). Go to each question. Then, place a check mark in the box next to the answer of your choice. The answers with the check marks are the ones that will count toward your score.

Now answer the main idea question. Follow the steps that are on the question page. Use a capital letter to mark your final answer to each part of the main idea question.

The Diagnostic Chart

Now move your final answers to the Diagnostic Chart on page 102. Use the column of boxes under number *1* for the answers to the first passage. Use the column of boxes under number *2* for the answers to the second passage, and so on.

Write the letter of your answer in the *upper* part of each block.

Correct your answers using the Answer Key on pages 100 and 101. When scoring your answers, do *not* use an *x* for *incorrect* or a *c* for *correct*. Instead, use this method. If your choice is correct, make no mark in the lower part of the answer block. If your choice is *in*correct, write the letter of the correct answer in the *lower* part of the block.

Thus, the answer column for each passage will show your incorrect answers. And it will also show the correct answers.

Your Total Comprehension Score

Go back to the passage you have just read. If you answered a question incorrectly, draw a line under the correct choice on the question page. Then write your score for each question in the circle provided. Add the scores to get your Total Comprehension Score.

Graphing Your Progress

After you have found your Total Comprehension Score, turn to the Progress Graph on page 103. Write your score in the box under the number for each passage. Then put an *x* along the line above the box to show your Total Comprehension Score. Join the *x*'s as you go. This will plot a line showing your progress.

Taking Corrective Action

Your incorrect answers give you a way to teach yourself how to read better. Take the time to study your wrong answers.

Go back to the question page. Read the correct answer (the one you have underlined) several times. With the correct answer in mind, go back to the passage itself. Read to see why the approved answer is better. Try to see where you made your mistake. Try to figure out why you chose a wrong answer.

The Steps in a Nutshell

Here's a quick review of the steps to follow. Following these steps is the way to get the most out of each *Essential Skills* book. Be sure you have read and understood all of the "To the Student" section on pages 11 through 22 before you start.

1. **Think About the Title of the Passage.** Try to get all the meaning the writer put into it.
2. **Read the Passage Quickly.**
3. **Answer the Questions, Using the Dot System.** Use dots to mark your unofficial answers. Don't look back at the passage.
4. **Read the Passage Again — Carefully.**
5. **Mark Your Final Answers.** Put a check mark (✓) in the box to note your final answer. Use capital letters for each part of the main idea question.
6. **Mark Your Answers on the Diagnostic Chart.** Record your final answers in the upper blocks of the chart on page 102.
7. **Correct Your Answers.** Use the Answer Key on pages 100 and 101. If an answer is not correct, (a) write the correct answer in the lower block, beneath your wrong answer. Then (b) go back to the question page. Place a line under the correct answer.
8. **Find Your Total Comprehension Score.** Find this by adding up the points you earned for each question.
9. **Graph Your Progress.** Mark and plot your scores on the graph on page 103.
10. **Take Corrective Action.** Read your wrong answers. Read the passage once more. Try to figure out why you were wrong.

Passages and Questions

1. A Gray Birch Is Born

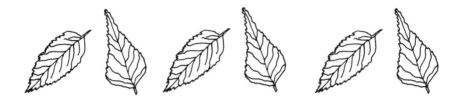

The seed from the gray birch was tiny. It was about the size of the *o*'s on this page. It had come loose, with many others like it, from the tree which grew at the edge of the forest next to an old field. A swift wind had bent and shaken the tall white trunk of the birch. Now the seed was sailing far out over the field. It was carried along by two little wings.

Other kinds of seeds had been blown from their trees by the same wind. But the seeds of the oak, beech and hickory trees were heavy nuts. They didn't have wings to carry them into the field. They had fallen to the forest floor a few feet (about a meter) from their parent trees.

The gust of wind blowing the birch seed began losing strength. Then the seed was falling! Below it the field was a jungle of grass and other plants. They had begun to grow in the field soon after the farmer had moved.

The tiny seed fell under a blackberry bush. Here it was quiet and shady. A few days later a light snow fell on the gray birch seed. All winter it lay still under the snow.

The early spring sun came through the blackberry stems. It cast long shadows on the melting snow. It took several days of warm weather to start the little seed growing. The seed sent tiny white roots into the dark soil where there should have been water and minerals. But there was little nourishment in the soil of the old field. Most of it had been used up by the crops which had grown there for many years. Other kinds of tree seedlings would have died in such poor soil. But the gray birch did not.

In a few months the seed had become a young tree. You might not think of it as a tree. The trunk was just about the thickness of a pencil lead. The tree had only eight leaves. But these green leaves were making food for the tree when the sun shone. They made the food out of carbon dioxide from the air and water brought up by the roots. This is called *photosynthesis* (fo to SIN thuh sis).

Time passed. On its first birthday the little tree was pushing its way up through the prickly stems of the blackberry bush. On its third birthday the gray birch was taller than the bush!

Each birthday that came found the gray birch taller. By its tenth year its trunk was about as thick as a baseball bat. The bark changed to a gray-white with V-shaped marks.

?

	Possible Score	Your Score

1. What would be another good title for this passage?

    ☐ a. Birth of a Tree
    ☐ b. How to Tell a Tree's Age
    ☐ c. Bears and Birch Trees
    ☐ d. Poems about Trees

(15) ◯

2. The food making process of green-leafed plants is called

    ☐ a. photographic.
    ☐ b. photoelectric.
    ☐ c. phototropic.
    ☐ d. photosynthesis.

(15) ◯

3. It seems that birch trees

    ☐ a. do not need soil that is rich in minerals.
    ☐ b. are easily killed by too much snow.
    ☐ c. do not lose their leaves in winter.
    ☐ d. have exploding seeds.

(15) ◯

4. A "jungle of grass" means the grass is

    ☐ a. a tropical kind.
    ☐ b. useful.
    ☐ c. very thick.
    ☐ d. well watered.

(15) ◯

5. As used in this passage, nourishment is

    ☐ a. wind.
    ☐ b. carbon dioxide.
    ☐ c. food.
    ☐ d. sunlight.

(15) ◯

6. Main Idea

	Answer	Score
Mark the main idea	M	⑩
Mark the statement that is a detail	D	⑤
Mark the statement that is too narrow	N	⑤
Mark the statement that is too broad	B	⑤

a. The gray birch becomes a hardy tree from a tiny seed.

b. Birch seeds are small and light enough to travel by wind.

c. Birches can grow where other trees would die.

d. Leaves use air and water to make their food.

Total Comprehension Score
(Add your scores and enter the total on the graph on page 103.)

Categories of Comprehension Questions

No. 1: Subject Matter	No. 4: Clarifying Devices
No. 2: Supporting Details	No. 5: Vocabulary in Context
No. 3: Conclusion	No. 6: Main Idea

2. A Gray Birch Grows Old

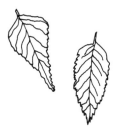

Each spring shiny birch leaves popped out from buds on the twigs. In a summer wind, they fluttered and danced on long stems. When autumn came, the leaves turned a deep gold color. The birch leaves fell each autumn. With the fallen leaves of the plants growing near it, they slowly built up a thin layer of rich soil.

One fall day, when the birch was twelve years old (that's almost middle age for a gray birch), a squirrel buried an acorn in the ground by the tree. The squirrel meant to come back for the acorn. But he forgot it.

After a time the acorn began to grow. It used minerals from the layer of rich soil that the birch and the other plants had laid down on top of the once bare soil. The leaves of the birch shaded the oak seedling from the hot sun.

The oak's growing close by didn't bother the birch for many years. Then one spring the birch flowered and opened its leaves for food. But the birch had trouble getting enough sunlight to make its food. The oak had grown too tall. Now oak leaves kept the sun from reaching the birch.

The next winter was a very hard one for all the birches. Heavy wet snow and thick coats of ice made them bend way over. Their top branches almost touched the ground. When it was younger, the gray birch would have sprung back up again when the snow and ice melted, but not this time! Somewhere in its thick trunk something had snapped. That spring the birch could not straighten up all the way.

Now insects were able to enter the weakened tree. Inside the trunk, they and their offspring ate away at the birch. It was also weakened by the woodpeckers that came to dig out the insects. The woodpeckers picked with their sharp bills and made a loud clatter.

The tiny seedlike spores of a fungus were carried to the tree by the wind. The spores entered the trunk through holes made by the insects. They sent out long thin threads into the wood. The fungus used the wood for food, too.

That winter a big storm toppled the gray birch to the ground. Snow covered it and rain fell upon it. Now other kinds of insects and fungi lived in the wood and used it for food. What was left became part of the soil after years had passed. Overhead the oak would go on growing for many more years, thanks to the birch.

?

		Possible Score	Your Score

1. This passage tells about

   ☐ a. gray birch seedlings.
   ☐ b. the roots and bark of a gray birch.
   ☐ c. the death of a gray birch.
   ☐ d. how gray birches get food.

   15   ◯

2. Each autumn the leaves of the birch became

   ☐ a. a deep gold.
   ☐ b. green.
   ☐ c. a brilliant red.
   ☐ d. orange.

   15   ◯

3. Rotting leaves

   ☐ a. can kill oak seedlings.
   ☐ b. poison the soil.
   ☐ c. add iron to the soil.
   ☐ d. make the soil rich.

   15   ◯

4. The woodpeckers that came to the birch were

   ☐ a. quiet.
   ☐ b. playful.
   ☐ c. noisy.
   ☐ d. bashful.

   15   ◯

5. A seedling is a

   ☐ a. bush.
   ☐ b. tree's trunk.
   ☐ c. fungus.
   ☐ d. young tree.

   15   ◯

6. Main Idea

	Answer	Score
Mark the main idea	M	(10)
Mark the statement that is a detail	D	(5)
Mark the statement that is too narrow	N	(5)
Mark the statement that is too broad	B	(5)

a. The fallen birch leaves helped make the soil rich. ☐ ◯

b. Survival of the fittest is the rule of all things in nature. ☐ ◯

c. Woodpeckers ate the insects which lived in the birch. ☐ ◯

d. As a gray birch ages and dies, it helps other plants to live. ☐ ◯

Total Comprehension Score
(Add your scores and enter the total on the graph on page 103.)

Categories of Comprehension Questions

No. 1: Subject Matter	No. 4: Clarifying Devices
No. 2: Supporting Details	No. 5: Vocabulary in Context
No. 3: Conclusion	No. 6: Main Idea

3. A Thing of Use and Beauty

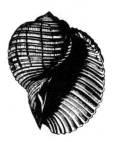

There are thousands of kinds of sea shells. They are found all over the world. They come in all sizes and shapes. The coquinas are as small as peas. The giant clam shell may be as large as three feet (about a meter) across. It may weigh 500 pounds (about 226.8 kilograms).

Through the years, shells have been put to many uses. They have been used as tools, ornaments and money. Many early peoples have used them for spoons, dishes, cups and even work tools. Today, tons of sea shells are ground to powder. Then the powder is used as lime to sweeten the soil of farms and gardens. This lime, too, is used to make a strong cement.

As ornaments, the shells may be made into strings of beads or earrings. They may be sewn onto a lady's dress. There was a time, not too long ago, when most of our buttons were made from the shells of the sea.

Shells have been used as money by the early people of lands the world over. *Wampum* was used by the North American Indians. It was nothing more than a string of matched shells.

The product of most value we get from shells is the white queen of the gem world, the pearl. Many divers have risked their lives for this warm, beautiful <u>orb</u>. Pearls are found chiefly in oysters. For three thousand years, the seas near Ceylon gave the world its best pearls. Now, Australia has earned that honor.

The sea shell has given much to people. But the greatest wonder that the sea shell gives is the wonder in the eyes of a child who holds a conch shell to his or her ear. Within it the child hears the ancient roll of the sea.

?

	Possible Score	Your Score

1. This passage tells us

   ☐ a. how sea shells are made.
   ☐ b. where to find giant clams.
   ☐ c. many facts about sea shells.
   ☐ d. how some shells got their name.

   Possible Score: (15)   Your Score: ○

2. Wampum was used as

   ☐ a. money.
   ☐ b. buttons.
   ☐ c. lime.
   ☐ d. tools.

   Possible Score: (15)   Your Score: ○

3. The author talks about pearls in order to suggest that

   ☐ a. pearls are easy to get.
   ☐ b. anyone can dive for pearls.
   ☐ c. experience is needed to locate pearls.
   ☐ d. diving for pearls is dangerous.

   Possible Score: (15)   Your Score: ○

4. The pearl is described as

   ☐ a. the most inexpensive gem.
   ☐ b. a mere sea shell.
   ☐ c. pure white.
   ☐ d. queen of the gem world.

   Possible Score: (15)   Your Score: ○

5. If something is shaped like an orb, it is

   ☐ a. square.
   ☐ b. bumpy.
   ☐ c. round.
   ☐ d. flat.

   Possible Score: (15)   Your Score: ○

6. Main Idea

	Answer	Score
Mark the main idea	M	⑩
Mark the statement that is a detail	D	⑤
Mark the statement that is too narrow	N	⑤
Mark the statement that is too broad	B	⑤

a. Sea shells are both beautiful and useful.

b. Australia has the best pearls in the world.

c. There are many uses for nature's products.

d. Shells are often used for ornaments.

Total Comprehension Score
(Add your scores and enter the
total on the graph on page 103.)

Categories of Comprehension Questions

No. 1: Subject Matter	No. 4: Clarifying Devices
No. 2: Supporting Details	No. 5: Vocabulary in Context
No. 3: Conclusion	No. 6: Main Idea

4. Finding Ancient Bugs

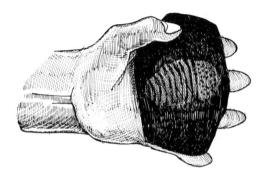

In Juab County, Utah, there is a mountain of ancient bugs. To find them you can start anywhere. Place your chisel in a crack in the side of the shale. Tap it with your hammer. The shale will fall open like the pages of a book. The bugs are sometimes very tiny. You have to look closely to see them. Check both sides of the stone before you crack open the next sheet. If you keep getting blank pages, move to another spot.

Sooner or later the shale will slice apart, and there will be a perfect rock bug large enough for you to see. It will be slightly raised and well <u>preserved</u>. Every line of its hard body armor will show clearly. It will have a flat, knobby head. It is called a *trilobite*. A good-sized trilobite will be from two to three inches (about 5.1 to 7.6 centimeters) long. But the tiny ones are to be treasured as well.

You might find a sheet nearly covered with them. They will be all sizes and facing in all directions. Other fossils might be mixed in with them. You might see swirly things that may be snails or worms. There could be little creatures whose shells look like butterfly wings. But most of them will be trilobites.

When you find a fossil sheet, you will want to take the whole piece. When you find a single bug, you can chip away some of the extra shale. You will then have less to carry.

The chipping has to be done with care. If the shale cracks across the middle, your bug may crack with it. Leave enough shale so you won't risk breaking a bug. You will crack a bug once in a while no matter how careful you are. But there will still be plenty of trilobites to take home. And plenty will remain in the gray mountain for others to find.

When you get home, you can have fun getting the bugs out of the shale. Let the shale soak in water for a few days, or as long as you want. Take a sheet out any time you feel like working on it. With your hammer and chisel tap gently around the edges of the bug. The water will have loosened it. You will be able to lift the trilobite out of the rock.

Now you can hold your stone bug in the palm of your hand. It will look almost like a real, live bug — as it was 500 million years ago.

?

	Possible Score	Your Score
1. What would be another good title for this passage?		

☐ a. Bugs For Sale
☐ b. Fossil Hunting
☐ c. Live Bugs Are the Best
☐ d. Nasty Pests

(15)   ◯

2. The mountain of bugs is made of

☐ a. shale.
☐ b. granite.
☐ c. marble.
☐ d. mica.

(15)   ◯

3. Trilobites

☐ a. were once small desert animals.
☐ b. had very soft bodies.
☐ c. are difficult to find.
☐ d. lived millions of years ago.

(15)   ◯

4. A "knobby head" is

☐ a. long.
☐ b. movable.
☐ c. round.
☐ d. soft.

(15)   ◯

5. A preserved bug has been well

☐ a. protected.
☐ b. fed.
☐ c. priced.
☐ d. discussed.

(15)   ◯

6. Main Idea

	Answer	Score
Mark the main idea	M	⑩
Mark the statement that is a detail	D	⑤
Mark the statement that is too narrow	N	⑤
Mark the statement that is too broad	B	⑤

a. A large trilobite will be 2–3 inches (about 5.1–7.6 centimeters) long.

b. Soak the shale in water for a few days to free the bug from the rock.

c. You can collect your own fossils.

d. Follow certain steps to get trilobite fossils from the mountain in Juab County.

Total Comprehension Score
(Add your scores and enter the total on the graph on page 103.)

Categories of Comprehension Questions

No. 1: Subject Matter	No. 4: Clarifying Devices
No. 2: Supporting Details	No. 5: Vocabulary in Context
No. 3: Conclusion	No. 6: Main Idea

5. Jack Is Back in Town

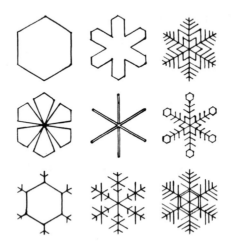

Frost does great harm to crops. But it also does some good. Some trees try to bear too much fruit. One or two frosts in the spring can nip off up to seventy-five percent of the blossoms. This lets the tree pour its strength into less, but better, fruit.

Around the time the fruit begins to ripen, it is Jack Frost who prods apple trees into putting a rich red bloom on their apples. With no frost to hurry the ripening along, the trees get a bit lazy. The trees then grow pale-looking apples, which are hard to sell.

You have heard of the harm done to highways by *frost heaves*. These cause the pavement to buckle and break. This isn't the same kind of frost you see on the lawn, but it's a first cousin. This kind of frost occurs when the ground gives up heat day after day. The earth freezes solid to a depth of four or five feet (about 1.2 or 1.5 meters). This swells the ground and breaks up roads.

But here, as in most things, there's always a brighter side. This same *frost action*, as it's called, loosens the soil for farmers and helps rot old crops. Thus, Jack Frost is breaking up roads. But he is also getting the soil ready for spring so farmers can grow bigger and better crops.

?

	Possible Score	Your Score

1. This passage describes mostly

   ☐ a. the way frost forms.
   ☐ b. the good and bad points of frost.
   ☐ c. how frost causes fruit to ripen.
   ☐ d. why frost is harmful.   (15)   ◯

2. When the ground freezes, the frost may go down

   ☐ a. 1 foot (about .3 meters).
   ☐ b. 4 or 5 feet (about 1.2 or 1.5 meters).
   ☐ c. 6 or 7 feet (about 1.8 or 2.1 meters).
   ☐ d. 10 feet (about 3.1 meters).   (15)   ◯

3. Without frost

   ☐ a. we would have poorer fruit.
   ☐ b. apples would be redder.
   ☐ c. your lawn would be thicker.
   ☐ d. farmers could grow bigger and better crops.   (15)   ◯

4. The phrase "but it's a first cousin" relates frost heaves to

   ☐ a. New England.
   ☐ b. the frost on your lawn.
   ☐ c. ice.
   ☐ d. the dew found on grass.   (15)   ◯

5. In this story, <u>prods</u> means

   ☐ a. damages.
   ☐ b. kills.
   ☐ c. stops.
   ☐ d. urges on.   (15)   ◯

6. Main Idea

	Answer	Score
Mark the main idea	M	(10)
Mark the statement that is a detail	D	(5)
Mark the statement that is too narrow	N	(5)
Mark the statement that is too broad	B	(5)

a. Trees may try to make too many fruits.

b. Frost can help as well as hurt.

c. There is good and bad in everything.

d. Frosts help farmers grow better crops.

Total Comprehension Score
(Add your scores and enter the total on the graph on page 103.)

Categories of Comprehension Questions

No. 1: Subject Matter	No. 4: Clarifying Devices
No. 2: Supporting Details	No. 5: Vocabulary in Context
No. 3: Conclusion	No. 6: Main Idea

6. Animal Baths

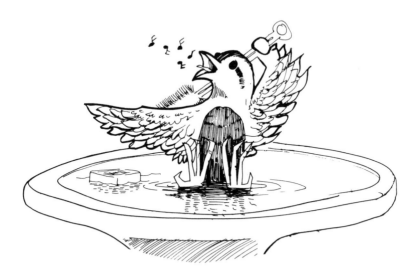

Most of you know that birds take baths. They might bathe in puddles, or in dust or sand holes, or in the snow. But there are many other kinds of animals that take "baths."

The vulture takes a sunbath in a treetop. Sitting on a high branch, it spreads its wings so sunshine can reach all its feathers. Vultures eat dead flesh. They pick up many germs on their bodies. The warm sun helps to kill the germs.

Kangaroo rats take sand baths. If you are in the desert where this tiny yellow-brown creature lives, you may see it rolling in the sand. As it rolls over and over, the sand acts as a brush to clean its fur.

Even the earthworm takes a bath. It does its bathing at night. When the earth is still and most animals are asleep, the worm crawls out of its underground home. It eats and drinks and takes a bath in the dew.

The elephant takes a shower. It <u>wades</u> out into the water. Then it sucks up water through its trunk and squirts it all over its body. If a baby elephant is near, it gets squirted, too.

But most animal mothers don't squirt their babies to get them clean. They lick them with their tongues. That's what a mother tiger does. Her tongue is rough and makes a good scrubber. She licks off any dirt that may be on her furry cub.

A cat uses its tongue as a "washcloth," too. Because its body is stretchy, it can reach most places with its tongue. The parts it can't reach it cleans in a different way. It wets its paw with its tongue and rubs it over its fur. Watch a pet cat do this when it washes its face.

No matter how an animal keeps clean, they all seem to know that a clean body is a healthy body.

?

	Possible Score	Your Score

1. This passage is about animals and how they

   ☐ a. dislike water.
   ☐ b. get dirty.
   ☐ c. treat their wounds.
   ☐ d. keep clean.

   15 ◯

2. Which animal likes to sit in the sun?

   ☐ a. The vulture
   ☐ b. The rat
   ☐ c. The elephant
   ☐ d. The tiger

   15 ◯

3. This passage suggests that to keep a body healthy one should

   ☐ a. be clean.
   ☐ b. get enough sleep.
   ☐ c. see a doctor.
   ☐ d. eat good food.

   15 ◯

4. In this passage, the elephant's trunk is like a

   ☐ a. cannon.
   ☐ b. shower.
   ☐ c. brush.
   ☐ d. weapon.

   15 ◯

5. The elephant <u>wades</u> into the water. This means the elephant

   ☐ a. kneels in the water.
   ☐ b. sits in the water.
   ☐ c. jumps into the water.
   ☐ d. walks into the water.

   15 ◯

6. Main Idea

	Answer	Score
Mark the main idea	M	(10)
Mark the statement that is a detail	D	(5)
Mark the statement that is too narrow	N	(5)
Mark the statement that is too broad	B	(5)

a. Many animals wash themselves with their tongues.

b. Animals take different kinds of baths to keep clean.

c. Vultures pick up many germs from the dead animals they eat.

d. Animals need to keep themselves clean.

Total Comprehension Score
(Add your scores and enter the total on the graph on page 103.)

Categories of Comprehension Questions

No. 1: Subject Matter	No. 4: Clarifying Devices
No. 2: Supporting Details	No. 5: Vocabulary in Context
No. 3: Conclusion	No. 6: Main Idea

7. What Do You Do if You Don't Have a Bathtub?

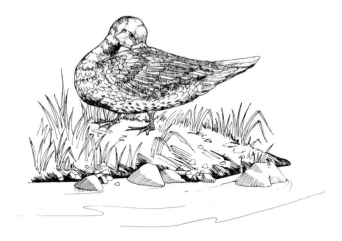

Animals like to keep themselves clean. Some of them even have a built-in "comb" to help them do the job right. Birds sometimes use their claws as combs. But more often they comb, or *preen,* themselves with their bills. As a matter of fact, they preen most of the day. Some birds run their bills over their feathers to make them lie in place. Their bills are often used to spread oil from a special gland. This waterproofs their feathers.

A hummingbird will clean its "comb" after it has used it. It will scrape and rub its beak with its claws until it is clean and shiny.

Insects have ways to keep clean, too. Bees have "combs" on their front legs with which they clean their antennae.

Ants have "brushes" on their "wrists" to scrub their antennae. They clean their antennae, then lick the "brushes" clean. They also lick their bodies with their tongues.

The queen ant has "ladies-in-waiting" that lick her clean. The "big boss" baboon is groomed by other baboons. They act as servants and pick their leader free of pests and dirt.

A sea creature which doesn't do the job itself is the fierce moray eel. It needs cleaning to rid its mouth of sea lice. So it swims to a reef in the ocean. Here small wrasses dart about. These little fish are not scared of the moray eel, no mater how <u>fierce</u> it may seem to others. In fact, the wrasses seem to be trying to get its notice. They seem to be calling out, "Here we are! At your service!" The eel opens its huge mouth, full of sharp teeth. Then some of the wrasses swim into it and start cleaning. When they are done, the eel just swims away.

Whether it is by splashing, rolling, squirting, licking, scratching or shaking, almost all animals have habits of cleanliness. They seem to know, just as people do, that one of the ways to stay healthy is to be clean.

	Possible Score	Your Score

1. This passage is mostly about how animals clean their

   ☐ a. nests.
   ☐ b. food.
   ☐ c. bodies.
   ☐ d. young.

   15   ○

2. How often do birds preen?

   ☐ a. Before eating
   ☐ b. Most of the day
   ☐ c. Once a day
   ☐ d. Twice a week

   15   ○

3. According to this passage

   ☐ a. preening can cause sickness.
   ☐ b. the moray eel is shy.
   ☐ c. very few animals keep clean.
   ☐ d. almost all animals practice cleanliness.

   15   ○

4. The writer talks about the queen ant, the "boss" baboon and the moray eel to show

   ☐ a. that some animals have servants clean them.
   ☐ b. how untidy some animals are.
   ☐ c. how splashing can clean animals.
   ☐ d. that some animals do not clean their young.

   15   ○

5. A <u>fierce</u> moray eel is

   ☐ a. calm.
   ☐ b. violent.
   ☐ c. shy.
   ☐ d. gentle.

   15   ○

6. Main Idea

	Answer	Score
Mark the main idea	M	(10)
Mark the statement that is a detail	D	(5)
Mark the statement that is too narrow	N	(5)
Mark the statement that is too broad	B	(5)

a. Some animals have others wash or clean them. ☐ ◯

b. Birds waterproof their feathers with oil. ☐ ◯

c. Many animals have unusual habits of cleanliness. ☐ ◯

d. Animals like to be clean. ☐ ◯

Total Comprehension Score
(Add your scores and enter the
total on the graph on page 103.)

Categories of Comprehension Questions

No. 1: Subject Matter	No. 4: Clarifying Devices
No. 2: Supporting Details	No. 5: Vocabulary in Context
No. 3: Conclusion	No. 6: Main Idea

8. The Ancient Comb

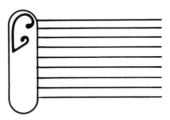

Today it costs a few cents to buy a comb for your hair. But 300 years ago, the comb was costly. It was then an important part of a person's wealth. Records show that pirates made it a point to take the combs of the people on board any ship they robbed.

How old are combs? Some combs, made of bone, have been found at the sites of early humans. This would place the comb's age at about 9,000 years. Even these combs were made to look pretty. They had shapes of animals carved on them.

The best combs of all were the ones that were used in church. Some of these combs were covered with gold. For a long time, it was a custom in the Greek Church to comb a priest's hair before all the people.

The comb is special to the Japanese. The Japanese women are known for the way they put up their thick, long, black hair. They hold their hair in place with combs. Some Japanese people feel that throwing away a comb will bring bad luck. Also, it is bad luck to pick one up. But a comb received as a parting gift is felt to bring good luck. The comb is supposed to make all the paths straight. This is because it makes one's hair straight.

It is not often that we stop to think about the history of things we use all the time. But if we did stop to think for a minute, then we would find that everything has its own history.

?

	Possible Score	Your Score

1. This passage is mostly about

   ☐ a. the Japanese combs.
   ☐ b. gold-plated combs.
   ☐ c. the history of combs.
   ☐ d. the cost of combs.

   15   ◯

2. The comb's age is about

   ☐ a. 200 years.
   ☐ b. 300 years.
   ☐ c. 2,000 years.
   ☐ d. 9,000 years.

   15   ◯

3. The comb has an

   ☐ a. unknown past.
   ☐ b. interesting history.
   ☐ c. unusual shape.
   ☐ d. odd name.

   15   ◯

4. The first paragraph shows that combs

   ☐ a. had different shapes.
   ☐ b. were expensive.
   ☐ c. could be very pretty.
   ☐ d. were interesting.

   15   ◯

5. A <u>costly</u> comb is one that is

   ☐ a. old.
   ☐ b. cheap.
   ☐ c. expensive.
   ☐ d. unknown.

   15   ◯

6. Main Idea

	Answer	Score
Mark the main idea	M	(10)
Mark the statement that is a detail	D	(5)
Mark the statement that is too narrow	N	(5)
Mark the statement that is too broad	B	(5)

a. Everything has its own history.

b. The comb's age is 9,000 years.

c. In its history, the comb went from rare and expensive to common and inexpensive.

d. Three hundred years ago, the comb was an important part of a person's wealth.

Total Comprehension Score
(Add your scores and enter the
total on the graph on page 103.)

Categories of Comprehension Questions

No. 1: Subject Matter	No. 4: Clarifying Devices
No. 2: Supporting Details	No. 5: Vocabulary in Context
No. 3: Conclusion	No. 6: Main Idea

9. Cypress Knees

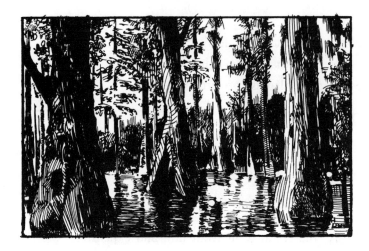

No one knows for sure the purpose of the strange knees of the cypress tree. Some botanists think that they help the tree to breathe. The cypress tree grows in the soft mud of the swamp. Its roots are in water-filled earth which contains little oxygen. Without oxygen the tree can't live. Perhaps bald cypress trees use these knees as "lungs." The knees might take in air and send it down to the roots of the tree.

But there are other scientists who think the purpose of the cypress knees is to help anchor the tree. Cypress roots are wide-spreading. Yet they do not grow deep enough to reach the solid earth. These people think that the knees act as a balance. The knees support the tall tree.

Bald cypresses can grow to be 75 to 200 feet (about 22.5 to 61 meters) tall. But they grow very slowly. One cypress tree, which is growing in Mexico, is thought to be close to 3,000 years old. This tree is 160 feet (about 48.8 meters) around at its base. It is 165 feet (about 49.5 meters) high.

The cypress tree is felt to be one of the best timber trees. The wood is light, but it is long lasting. Cypress wood is often known as *wood everlasting.*

In early spring the bald cypress grows loose clusters of small cones. Pollen falls from some of these cones into other small cones and fertilizes them. The cones that have caught the pollen stay on the tree and grow. Inside these cones are thin, flat seeds that are about a half inch (about 1.3 centimeters) long. When they are ripe, the seeds fall.

If the seed falls in a swamp and grows, it will be a tree that has the strange knees. But if the seed should land on dry earth and grow, it will be a tree that does not have knees. When a cypress swamp is drained, the knees rot away. But the trees do not die.

	Possible Score	Your Score

1. What would be another good title for this passage?

   ☐ a. Plants of the Swamp
   ☐ b. Trees and Knees
   ☐ c. Uses of the Cypress Tree
   ☐ d. Cypress Fertilizer

   (15)   ◯

2. According to this passage, in order to live the cypress tree needs

   ☐ a. nitrogen.
   ☐ b. carbon dioxide.
   ☐ c. hydrogen.
   ☐ d. oxygen.

   (15)   ◯

3. Cypress wood

   ☐ a. rots easily.
   ☐ b. is useful.
   ☐ c. is worthless.
   ☐ d. has a poor quality.

   (15)   ◯

4. The third paragraph tells us that cypress trees

   ☐ a. produce cones.
   ☐ b. are very valuable.
   ☐ c. grow very fast.
   ☐ d. live a long time.

   (15)   ◯

5. Timber is

   ☐ a. wood used in building.
   ☐ b. a cone-producing tree.
   ☐ c. wood that cannot be cut.
   ☐ d. shrubbery.

   (15)   ◯

6. Main Idea

	Answer	Score
Mark the main idea	M	(10)
Mark the statement that is a detail	D	(5)
Mark the statement that is too narrow	N	(5)
Mark the statement that is too broad	B	(5)

a. Cypress trees may live to be several thousand years old.

b. Cypress knees help cypress grow in swamps, but no one knows how.

c. Some cypress trees have knees, and some do not.

d. The knees of a cypress may help to balance the tall tree.

Total Comprehension Score
(Add your scores and enter the total on the graph on page 103.)

Categories of Comprehension Questions

No. 1: Subject Matter	No. 4: Clarifying Devices
No. 2: Supporting Details	No. 5: Vocabulary in Context
No. 3: Conclusion	No. 6: Main Idea

10. Flying Frogs

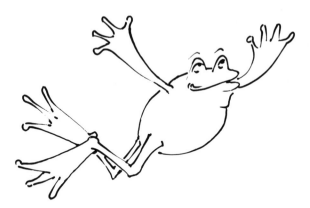

In a tropical forest somewhere in Asia, a small tree frog leaps into the air. But it leaps from high up in a tree! First, it arches its body. Then it spreads out the wide webbing between its fingers and toes and leaps. Down it glides through the air. It reaches the limb of a tree thirty-five feet (about 10.7 meters) away.

The flying frog leaps from branch to branch. In this way, it catches flying insects that it must have for its daily food. Then the frog grows tired. It sits down on a limb and waits for the insects to fly by.

The tree frog has large, bulging eyes. They peer out well above its broad head. The frog can see in front, behind, above and to both sides — all at the same time. Once in a while, though, a flying tree frog is caught off guard by a hunting tree snake or a bird and eaten.

All tree frogs have flat sticky discs on the tips of their toes. But flying tree frogs have discs that are huge compared to the size of their bodies. When this frog goes gliding through the air, it needs to push just one toe-disc against a tree branch. It can then hang on quite safely. Little glands spread the sticky substance, like glue or tape, over the discs. The frog can go straight up the side of a tree. It can walk on the underside of a limb and not fall off. It won't leave sticky footprints behind either!

One kind of tree frog lives in Borneo. This one glides through the air on webbed feet that spread out to a size greater than its body. Another kind in southern China and in parts of Malaya is large and bright in color. People there worship it as a god. It is carried around on a sacred chair.

?

	Possible Score	Your Score

1. This passage is about

☐ a. the leopard frog.
☐ b. pickerel frogs.
☐ c. frogs and toads.
☐ d. tree frogs.

(15)   ◯

2. Most flying frogs eat

☐ a. meat.
☐ b. insects.
☐ c. grass.
☐ d. moss.

(15)   ◯

3. To some people in China and Malaya, the frog is

☐ a. a good luck sign.
☐ b. a special treat.
☐ c. thought to be evil.
☐ d. part of their religion.

(15)   ◯

4. To be "caught off guard" means to be

☐ a. well prepared.
☐ b. warned.
☐ c. surprised.
☐ d. attacked.

(15)   ◯

5. A sacred chair is

☐ a. holy.
☐ b. sticky.
☐ c. huge.
☐ d. expensive.

(15)   ◯

6. Main Idea

	Answer	Score
Mark the main idea	M	(10)
Mark the statement that is a detail	D	(5)
Mark the statement that is too narrow	N	(5)
Mark the statement that is too broad	B	(5)

a. Some creatures seem to be able to fly.

b. Small glands spread the sticky substance over the flying frog's toe-discs.

c. Some tree frogs can fly by gliding through the air.

d. The flying frog of Borneo glides on large webbed feet.

Total Comprehension Score
(Add your scores and enter the total on the graph on page 103.)

Categories of Comprehension Questions

No. 1: Subject Matter	No. 4: Clarifying Devices
No. 2: Supporting Details	No. 5: Vocabulary in Context
No. 3: Conclusion	No. 6: Main Idea

11. Keep Off My Farm

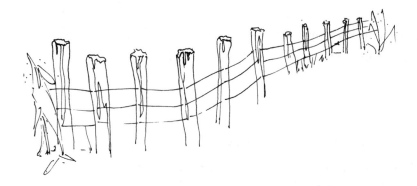

Hunters are not welcome on my farm. I can get by without them. Here's why: I used to let hunters shoot rabbits and pheasants on my place. But, no more. I got sick and tired of a few "sporting" people who just didn't care what they did. All the bad things you can think of, they did. They left open a gate. So my cows got into another field. My kids have been insulted with foul language. Fires have been set in my woods. I've found my fences smashed down or cut. One hunter bragged about carrying a pair of pliers so he wouldn't have to climb a fence.

How would you like to have an <u>expensive</u> machine fouled up by beer cans? The cans are thrown on the ground by careless hunters. Wouldn't you be mad to have to shoo your kids in the house because shotgun pellets were rattling on the roof and off the walls of your home? Would you like to have your livestock stampeded by dogs? My livestock have even been shot at. City slickers can't tell the difference between a game animal and a prize boar or a dairy cow!

Sporting? No! Too many of them care only about their own pleasure. They don't think about the rights of others.

What would make me change my mind? Well, I'd like to see some of these eager beavers show up at haying time to ask if they could lend a hand! Or maybe they could come out to ask if they could help me with the chores. They could invite me for a weekend in the city. It ought to be a two-way street. When all hunters are good sports, then I'll welcome them once more.

	Possible Score	Your Score

1. What would be another good title for this passage?

   ☐ a. A Hunting Farm That Works
   ☐ b. Big Game for Big Hunters
   ☐ c. To Hunt or Not to Hunt
   ☐ d. Not *All* Hunters Are Good Sports

   Possible Score: (15)   Your Score: ◯

2. The hunters in this passage were mainly after

   ☐ a. quail and fox.
   ☐ b. rabbits and pheasants.
   ☐ c. doves and quail.
   ☐ d. beaver and muskrat.

   Possible Score: (15)   Your Score: ◯

3. We can see that some hunters are

   ☐ a. thoughtless.
   ☐ b. generous.
   ☐ c. considerate.
   ☐ d. kind.

   Possible Score: (15)   Your Score: ◯

4. A "careless hunter" is

   ☐ a. cautious.
   ☐ b. showy.
   ☐ c. reckless.
   ☐ d. careful.

   Possible Score: (15)   Your Score: ◯

5. An expensive machine is

   ☐ a. cheap.
   ☐ b. broken.
   ☐ c. easy to run.
   ☐ d. costly.

   Possible Score: (15)   Your Score: ◯

6. Main Idea

	Answer	Score
Mark the main idea	M	(10)
Mark the statement that is a detail	D	(5)
Mark the statement that is too narrow	N	(5)
Mark the statement that is too broad	B	(5)

a. Hunters sometimes cause trouble. ☐ ○

b. A beer can may damage a farm machine. ☐ ○

c. Careless hunters sometimes shoot livestock. ☐ ○

d. Selfish hunters are poor "sports" to farmers. ☐ ○

Total Comprehension Score
(Add your scores and enter the
total on the graph on page 103.)

Categories of Comprehension Questions

No. 1: Subject Matter	No. 4: Clarifying Devices
No. 2: Supporting Details	No. 5: Vocabulary in Context
No. 3: Conclusion	No. 6: Main Idea

12. Sleep Tight

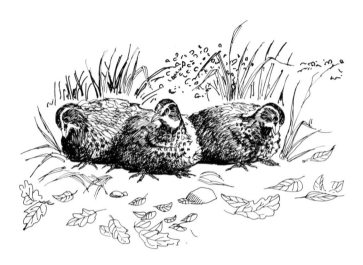

You bed down under warm blankets on a cold winter night. Do you ever wonder where animals sleep when cold winds blow? Many wild creatures such as chipmunks, bears, turtles, frogs and some snakes hibernate or sleep through the winter. But what about deer, raccoons, gray squirrels and winter birds? Where do they sleep? How do they keep warm with just fur or feathers to protect them?

On some cold days, gray squirrels can be seen on the ground. Other days there aren't any squirrels in sight. They are asleep in their nests high up in tall trees. Their nests are big, bulky balls of leaves and twigs in the forks of trees.

Wild rabbits doze through the day, too. They like to sleep in shallow holes in the ground. They like best the holes where dry weed-stalks stand all winter. Other rabbits crawl into old groundhog holes to nap.

Naturalists wanted to find a raccoon's winter sleeping place. They searched for some time. Then they found a raccoon asleep in an empty hawk's nest high in a tree.

Out in the woods, birds, such as quail, gather into tight huddles on the cold ground. They keep warm this way. Their tails touch each other like spokes in a wheel. Their heads point outward.

Grouse like to sit in pines or hemlocks, or in tangles of grapevines. When snow is on the ground, grouse will back into the snow. Sometimes they fly headfirst into a white drift! Their body heat makes a small "instant" burrow.

If you should come upon a sleeping bat, you will see it with wings folded, hanging upside down. Bats like dark caves or the eaves of an old barn.

Bats, birds or bunnies — don't worry about the wild creatures. They may be warmer than you — even on the coldest night.

	Possible Score	Your Score

1. This passage tells us

   ☐ a. about animal fur.
   ☐ b. how feathers help to hold heat in.
   ☐ c. where animals go to keep warm.
   ☐ d. the kinds of food animals eat to stay warm.

   15

2. During winter months, frogs and snakes

   ☐ a. grow a thicker skin.
   ☐ b. hibernate.
   ☐ c. hunt more food.
   ☐ d. nest near water.

   15

3. The grouse seems to make a burrow in the snow by using

   ☐ a. a thick cover of leaves.
   ☐ b. his body heat to melt it.
   ☐ c. bits of animals fur.
   ☐ d. nearby sticks to sweep it aside.

   15

4. The writer mentions the quail to show that some birds

   ☐ a. gather together to keep warm.
   ☐ b. grow thicker feathers.
   ☐ c. hibernate.
   ☐ d. fly into snow drifts to make burrows.

   15

5. Naturalists study mostly

   ☐ a. rocks.
   ☐ b. types of soil.
   ☐ c. animals and plants.
   ☐ d. weather.

   15

6. Main Idea

	Answer	Score
Mark the main idea	M	10
Mark the statement that is a detail	D	5
Mark the statement that is too narrow	N	5
Mark the statement that is too broad	B	5

a. Wild birds and animals must protect themselves from the weather.

b. Wild birds and animals have different ways of staying warm during winter.

c. Bats sleep hanging upside down in dark caves or eaves of old barns.

d. Squirrels build nests of leaves and twigs to keep them warm on cold days.

Total Comprehension Score
(Add your scores and enter the total on the graph on page 103.)

Categories of Comprehension Questions

No. 1: Subject Matter	No. 4: Clarifying Devices
No. 2: Supporting Details	No. 5: Vocabulary in Context
No. 3: Conclusion	No. 6: Main Idea

13. The Ocean Forest

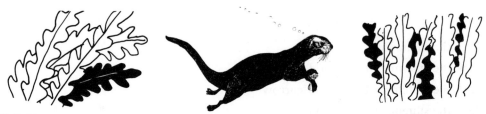

Want to visit the home of the sea otters? Then think of a woods with no trees, birds or deer. Instead there are huge seaweeds (called *kelp*), sea stars, crabs, fish — and the otters.

Kelp is a kind of alga. Kelp is anchored to the ocean floor by rootlike *holdfasts* that cling to large rocks. Stems, or *stipes,* grow in a thick clump from each holdfast. The stipes grow up to the surface. They can grow as far as 130 feet (about 39 meters) from the bottom!

Giant kelp can grow as much as two feet (about .61 meters) in length a day. This plant is the fastest growing in the world. Each of its leaves has a bulb filled with gas. These bulbs keep the leaves afloat on the surface in the sun. The sun is needed by the kelp plant. The kelp makes its food from the sun.

A kelp forest looks like a tall apartment building with tenants living on many floors. Sea stars, lobsters and crabs crawl on the bottom looking for food. They also use the plants as places to hide. Fish, shrimp and snails live in the middle. Sea otters spend most of their time at the top.

The sea forest has its share of problems. The strong waves of a storm may uproot the kelp plants. They then wash up on shore where they die. But the forest's worst problem is the spiny animal that looks like a crawling pincushion — the *sea urchin*. These urchins mostly eat kelp blades that fall to the bottom. But sometimes there are too many urchins. Then they start to nibble on the stipes. This causes the stipes to break and float away and die.

The sea otter is the forest's best defense against sea urchins. Otters love to feed on urchins. But eating them isn't easy. The sea otter must first dive as deep as thirty-three feet (about 9.9 meters) to search for them. It has only about a minute to look before it must go up for more air. When the otter finds a sea urchin, it grabs the urchin and a rock. Yes, a rock! The otter grabs the sea urchin in one front paw. It tucks the rock under its other front paw. The otter swims to the surface. It rolls on its back and puts the rock on its chest. It bangs the urchin on the rock until its shell cracks. The otter's tough little paws are not harmed by the urchin's stinging spines.

The sea otter is a big eater. It can eat about one-fifth of its own body weight in food each day. Zoo keepers say that in a zoo they can eat more than a lion does!

The sea otter's stomach is now full. Its fur is clean and <u>groomed</u>. Now it wraps kelp around its body. It then goes to sleep. It won't worry about drifting away from its home in the sea forest because the kelp holds it.

?

	Possible Score	Your Score

1. The ocean forest is made up mostly of

   ☐ a. turtle grass.
   ☐ b. giant seaweed.
   ☐ c. lichens.
   ☐ d. rocks and underwater caves.

   15   ◯

2. Kelp is a kind of

   ☐ a. fungus.
   ☐ b. moss.
   ☐ c. plankton.
   ☐ d. alga.

   15   ◯

3. We can guess that

   ☐ a. without the sea otter the ocean forest would be greatly damaged.
   ☐ b. underwater forests have become so thick that they are killing many small fish.
   ☐ c. pollution causes seaweed to grow.
   ☐ d. sea urchins are dangerous and can kill a sea otter.

   15   ◯

4. The sea urchin is a "crawling pincushion." This means the sea urchin

   ☐ a. can pick up sharp objects.
   ☐ b. is easily wounded.
   ☐ c. is soft and fleshy.
   ☐ d. has sharp spines.

   15   ◯

5. Groomed fur is

   ☐ a. dull.
   ☐ b. neat.
   ☐ c. oily.
   ☐ d. dirty.

   15   ◯

6. Main Idea

	Answer	Score
Mark the main idea	M	(10)
Mark the statement that is a detail	D	(5)
Mark the statement that is too narrow	N	(5)
Mark the statement that is too broad	B	(5)

a. Sea otters live in kelp forests.

b. The kelp forest and the sea otter help each other to live.

c. All living things depend on one another.

d. Sea otters use a rock to break open the sea urchins they eat.

Total Comprehension Score
(Add your scores and enter the total on the graph on page 103.)

Categories of Comprehension Questions

No. 1: Subject Matter	No. 4: Clarifying Devices
No. 2: Supporting Details	No. 5: Vocabulary in Context
No. 3: Conclusion	No. 6: Main Idea

14. The Squirrel's Helpers

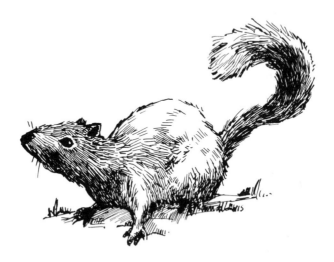

The gray squirrel is the one with the bushy tail. It lives in the woods with the red and flying squirrels. It is nearly twice as big as its cousin the red squirrel.

This squirrel uses its great gray brush of a tail in many ways. It whisks its tail ahead of it when it is in a place it does not know. It jerks it back and forth while it eats. In both cases it is a decoy. An enemy would attack the moving tail, not the squirrel itself! This squirrel takes flying leaps or runs on narrow limbs. So it also uses its great tail to balance itself. Should the limb break, its tail acts as a parachute to slow its fall.

Many animals try to catch squirrels. So the squirrels need ways to protect themselves. They have many defenses. They can escape owls and foxes by being on the alert. They must be ready to dash up a tree and into a hole. They can fit in holes too small for a weasel to squeeze through. A snake might climb up to the nest. The parent squirrels will attack and bite it to make it go away.

I once saw a red squirrel run under a brush pile when a hawk flew near. At the same time, a gray squirrel flattened itself against the trunk of a big gum tree. The hawk alighted on a dead pine branch. It looked around for five minutes while I sat hidden and watched.

The two squirrels moved not a hair. Flapping its great wings, the hawk took off. It passed within six feet of the gray squirrel. But the squirrel's gray and white fur blended with the gray and white bark of the gum. The hawk couldn't see it.

Soon the gray squirrel twitched its tail and ran on up the tree. And, with a lively chirrup, the red squirrel bounced out from its brush pile hiding place to finish eating its pine cone.

?

	Possible Score	Your Score

1. This passage tells us how gray squirrels

   ☐ a. protect themselves.
   ☐ b. mate.
   ☐ c. care for their families.
   ☐ d. find food.

   (15)   ◯

2. A close cousin of the gray squirrel is

   ☐ a. the red fox.
   ☐ b. the red squirrel.
   ☐ c. the woodchuck.
   ☐ d. the weasel.

   (15)   ◯

3. The gray squirrel seems to be very

   ☐ a. careless.
   ☐ b. alert.
   ☐ c. lazy.
   ☐ d. mean.

   (15)   ◯

4. The tail of the gray squirrel can be described as

   ☐ a. unnecessary.
   ☐ b. worthless.
   ☐ c. useful.
   ☐ d. troublesome.

   (15)   ◯

5. As used in this passage, <u>alighted</u> means

   ☐ a. landed.
   ☐ b. missed.
   ☐ c. fell.
   ☐ d. flew away.

   (15)   ◯

6. Main Idea

	Answer	Score
Mark the main idea	M	⑩
Mark the statement that is a detail	D	⑤
Mark the statement that is too narrow	N	⑤
Mark the statement that is too broad	B	⑤

a. The gray squirrel can hide by staying very still.

b. Squirrels survive the forest dangers in many ways.

c. Squirrels use their tails for balance when they run or leap.

d. Squirrels have many natural aids for protection and safety.

Total Comprehension Score
(Add your scores and enter the total on the graph on page 103.)

Categories of Comprehension Questions

No. 1: Subject Matter	No. 4: Clarifying Devices
No. 2: Supporting Details	No. 5: Vocabulary in Context
No. 3: Conclusion	No. 6: Main Idea

15. Quizzy

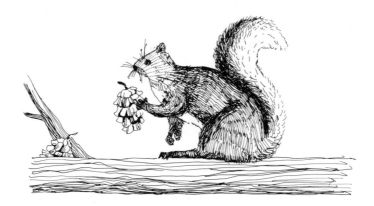

On my walks, I came across another kind of squirrel. This was the red squirrel. I saw that the red squirrels are bigger than the flying squirrels. It is this squirrel which takes over the woods when the small flying acrobats have gone to rest for the day.

The red squirrel is full of chatter. It is quite a lively creature. It likes to eat pine or spruce cones. It picks these apart to get at the seeds. I would find pieces of cone in small piles.

Like the gray and flying squirrels, the red squirrel stores food for winter. But it stores more than the others do.

Have you ever seen a pine cone wedged in the crotch of a maple? Most likely a red squirrel put it there to dry. As it dries, it opens. It can then get at the seeds with ease.

Is that a mushroom high in the twigs of a dogwood? It, too, is being dried before it is stored away in a hollow tree, under a stump or in an empty birds' nest.

I've had fun watching Quizzy, the inquisitive red squirrel whom I fed for three winters in the woods. I would place corn, peanuts and pastry on a log. Then I sat at one end, waiting for Quizzy to come to the other. She soon got used to me. Often she looked up into my face and chirped. She seemed to ask if I were safe to be near. To keep her from being afraid, I never tried to touch her. I just let her come and go.

After eating her fill, Quizzy stored what was left. She buried whole nuts in the forest floor. She carried nutmeats, bread and pastry high up the trees to stuff into cracks or behind loose bark. She moved a whole sweet potato away by pushing it in front of her. She ran ahead now and then to poke sticks out of the way or to bite off twigs which were in her path. But no matter what Quizzy did, I was delighted by her.

	Possible Score	Your Score

1. Quizzy is a

   ☐ a. gray squirrel.
   ☐ b. flying squirrel.
   ☐ c. red squirrel.
   ☐ d. ground squirrel.

   (15)   ◯

2. Quizzy liked to eat

   ☐ a. pesty insects.
   ☐ b. grass seeds.
   ☐ c. acorns.
   ☐ d. pine or spruce cones.

   (15)   ◯

3. After reading this passage, we can see that during winter months some animals

   ☐ a. live off the food they have stored.
   ☐ b. bury themselves in a deep burrow.
   ☐ c. grow thick fur coats.
   ☐ d. begin to hibernate.

   (15)   ◯

4. The writer of this story thinks of Quizzy as a

   ☐ a. pest.
   ☐ b. danger.
   ☐ c. science experiment.
   ☐ d. pet.

   (15)   ◯

5. An <u>inquisitive</u> squirrel is

   ☐ a. curious.
   ☐ b. smart.
   ☐ c. lazy.
   ☐ d. quiet.

   (15)   ◯

6. Main Idea

	Answer	Score
Mark the main idea	M	10
Mark the statement that is a detail	D	5
Mark the statement that is too narrow	N	5
Mark the statement that is too broad	B	5

a. In their forest home, squirrels store food to live on.

b. A red squirrel will store mushrooms, pine cones and even sweet potatoes.

c. Red squirrels like to pull pine or spruce cones apart to eat the seeds.

d. Red squirrels dry and store as much food as they can get.

Total Comprehension Score
(Add your scores and enter the total on the graph on page 103.)

Categories of Comprehension Questions

No. 1: Subject Matter	No. 4: Clarifying Devices
No. 2: Supporting Details	No. 5: Vocabulary in Context
No. 3: Conclusion	No. 6: Main Idea

16. The Art of Make-up

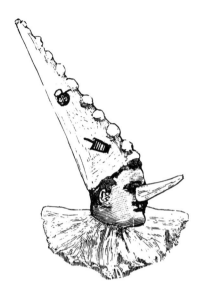

As the stage lights dim, we see an old man. He is broken and empty, with bent back, close to death. We feel the pain in his measured limp and sit forward tensely in the dark. His eyebrows bristle above eyes that are barely more than sockets of dead flame. His craggy nose is moist with tears. Breath by breath his life runs out. The curtain falls.

After a long span of silence, our wonder gathers into waves of applause. In a short while we go out into the night. But the face and anguish of a man we did not know three hours before is burned into our minds.

Backstage, the "old man" flings off his padded hump. He peels away his clay nose, his crepe-hair beard and his gray wig. He sinks his fingers into a large jar. He washes neck and cheeks, forehead and ears with the smooth, cool cream. With a soft towel he wipes the grease and pigment from his face. It is a face just thirty-three years old. Friends crowd into his dressing room to congratulate him.

The next evening, an hour before curtain time, the dressing room is silent. The actor lays out his sticks of grease paint on the make-up table. He ties a shoulder cover around his neck and begins the whole process all over again. With a skilled hand, he puts on the make-up which will change him into somebody else.

?

	Possible Score	Your Score

1. What would be another good title for this passage?

   ☐ a. New Ways to Apply Make-up
   ☐ b. Different Kinds of Make-up
   ☐ c. How Make-up Can Change You   (15)   ◯
   ☐ d. The History of Make-up

2. How long does it take this actor to put on make-up?

   ☐ a. 45 minutes
   ☐ b. About 1 hour
   ☐ c. 1½ hours   (15)   ◯
   ☐ d. 2 hours

3. This passage suggests that

   ☐ a. some actors are skilled at putting on their own make-up.
   ☐ b. all young actors take the parts of "old men."
   ☐ c. acting is an easy job.   (15)   ◯
   ☐ d. putting make-up on is fun.

4. The first two paragraphs of this passage

   ☐ a. explain make-up.
   ☐ b. show how to use make-up.
   ☐ c. make the reader laugh.   (15)   ◯
   ☐ d. make the reader feel he or she is at the theater.

5. Another word for <u>pigment</u> would be

   ☐ a. hair.
   ☐ b. color.
   ☐ c. charcoal.   (15)   ◯
   ☐ d. scars.

6. Main Idea

	Answer	Score
Mark the main idea	M	(10)
Mark the statement that is a detail	D	(5)
Mark the statement that is too narrow	N	(5)
Mark the statement that is too broad	B	(5)

a. Actors use make-up to change themselves into the characters they play.

b. An actor uses cream to remove make-up.

c. A man can change how he looks with make-up.

d. An actor becomes an old man by using make-up, a beard and a wig.

Total Comprehension Score
(Add your scores and enter the total on the graph on page 103.)

Categories of Comprehension Questions

No. 1: Subject Matter	No. 4: Clarifying Devices
No. 2: Supporting Details	No. 5: Vocabulary in Context
No. 3: Conclusion	No. 6: Main Idea

17. Tricky Tongues

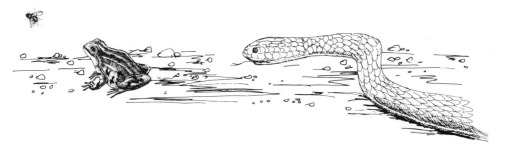

Some animals wouldn't have food if it weren't for their tongues. Their tongues are their best tool for getting food. And they use their tongues to "handle" food as they chew and swallow.

Snakes use their tongues to find prey. A snake often flicks its tongue out. In this way, it picks up odors from the air and ground. When it draws in its tongue, it places it in or near two pits. The pits are called *Jacobson's organ* and are in the roof of the snake's mouth. These pits do the same job your nose does — they smell. So, thanks to its tongue, a snake can follow the scent of an animal.

Once a snake has caught its prey and begins to swallow, it no longer needs the tongue. It just slips its tongue into a pocket on the floor of its mouth.

Geckos are a kind of lizard. They use their tongues for picking up and gulping their insect prey. Also, their see-through eyelids get dirty. So the geckos can flip up their tongues and wipe the lids clean.

Most animals' tongues are attached at the back of the mouth. But the tongues of all frogs and toads are attached at the front. They can shoot their sticky tongues forward to catch unsuspecting insects.

The stars of this shooting tongue parade are the chameleons. Their tongues reach quite a distance. Their tongues are as long as their body and tail. Spying an insect with its bulging eyes, a chameleon slowly moves into striking range. In a flash — faster than your eye can see — the chameleon zips out its tongue and snares the prey with the sticky tip. It pulls it back into its mouth.

Where to keep this long tongue is no problem for the chameleon. When not using it, the chameleon folds it up like a jack-in-the-box.

The anteater would never get enough ants and termites by picking them up one at a time. It has to get food in king-sized amounts. And its tongue helps it do this with ease.

An anteater may search for ant and termite nests hour after hour. When it finds one, it tears the nest apart with its sharp front claws. Then it jabs into the nest with a tongue two feet (about .60 meters) long. The insects stick by the hundreds! They stick to it because the tongue is coated with gluelike saliva. An anteater's tongue gets a new coating of saliva each time it draws the tongue back into its mouth. And so it prepares for the next hunt with its tricky tongue.

	Possible Score	Your Score

1. What would be another good title for this passage?

  ☐ a. How Does the Tongue Taste?
  ☐ b. Uses for Tricky Tongues
  ☐ c. Forked Tongues Are Best
  ☐ d. Animals Without Tongues

Possible Score 15 — **Your Score** ◯

2. A gecko is a kind of

  ☐ a. toad.
  ☐ b. frog.
  ☐ c. snake.
  ☐ d. lizard.

15 ◯

3. Without their tongues, some animals

  ☐ a. could not hear.
  ☐ b. would certainly starve.
  ☐ c. could not mate.
  ☐ d. would find it difficult to sleep.

15 ◯

4. A see-through eyelid is

  ☐ a. clear.
  ☐ b. stained.
  ☐ c. dark.
  ☐ d. cloudy.

15 ◯

5. An <u>unsuspecting</u> insect is

  ☐ a. very large.
  ☐ b. well hidden.
  ☐ c. hungry.
  ☐ d. easily surprised.

15 ◯

	Answer	Score
Mark the main idea	M	(10)
Mark the statement that is a detail	D	(5)
Mark the statement that is too narrow	N	(5)
Mark the statement that is too broad	B	(5)

a. A snake can follow its prey by smelling the trail with its tongue.

b. Animals must obtain their own food to survive.

c. Several animals use their tongues as a tool for getting food.

d. A chameleon has a tongue which is as long as its body and tail.

Total Comprehension Score
(Add your scores and enter the
total on the graph on page 103.)

Categories of Comprehension Questions

No. 1: Subject Matter	No. 4: Clarifying Devices
No. 2: Supporting Details	No. 5: Vocabulary in Context
No. 3: Conclusion	No. 6: Main Idea

18. The Quaking Aspen

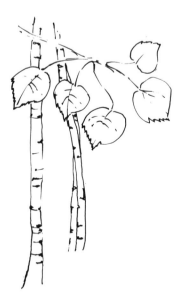

Everything seems to be against the quaking aspen tree. If its ripe seeds do not sprout in three weeks, they die. Some seeds do fall on moist soil and sprout. But the sprouts are often eaten by ants or <u>withered</u> by fungi. Quaking aspens which are a year old have tender bark. The bark makes a good meal for a hungry meadow mouse or snowshoe hare. Saplings as tall as you are seem to taste great to mule deer, white-tailed deer and moose. In summer, cutworms and sawflies chew the bright green leaves.

When life is that tough for a tree, you'd think it would give up. As with most trees, some quaking aspens survive in spite of their problems. They are found in more places in our country than any other tree!

These great trees are called *pioneers*. They are very good pioneers, too! Quaking aspens can grow where most other trees can't. They flourish on land that is burned or strip-mined. They can even grow where it is barren of all other plants.

Like most other pioneer trees, these aspens are tops in the seed business. Just one tree can produce millions of seeds. Each seed comes with its own parachute. The seeds sail away on the wind.

Seeds that drift into an open place and find a bit of moist soil will quickly sprout. In a few years there are tall saplings which send out roots. From these roots other saplings can sprout. They grow up through the weeds and brush to become new trees. As they grow, they crowd other plants aside. Soon they make enough shade and soak up enough water to kill the weeds and brush under them. The quaking aspens have then won a battle.

	Possible Score	Your Score

1. This passage is about the quaking aspen and how it

    ☐ a. sheds its bark.
    ☐ b. is cut.
    ☐ c. grows.   (15)   ◯
    ☐ d. survived the winter.

2. The seeds of the aspen are scattered by

    ☐ a. humans.
    ☐ b. animals.
    ☐ c. water.
    ☐ d. wind.   (15)   ◯

3. Aspens are called "pioneers" because they

    ☐ a. are an experiment.
    ☐ b. grow where most trees cannot.
    ☐ c. are a new kind of tree.   (15)   ◯
    ☐ d. grow only in thick woods.

4. The first paragraph tells us the kind of things that

    ☐ a. help aspens grow.
    ☐ b. ecologists use to study trees.
    ☐ c. kill aspens.   (15)   ◯
    ☐ d. aspens are used for.

5. A <u>withered</u> tree is

    ☐ a. green and thick.
    ☐ b. brown and tan.
    ☐ c. shriveled and dried.
    ☐ d. big and tough.   (15)   ◯

6. Main Idea

<table>
<tr><td></td><td></td><td>**Answer**</td><td>**Score**</td></tr>
<tr><td>Mark the main idea</td><td>. . . . .</td><td>M</td><td>(10)</td></tr>
<tr><td>Mark the statement that is a detail</td><td>. . . . .</td><td>D</td><td>(5)</td></tr>
<tr><td>Mark the statement that is too narrow</td><td>. . . . .</td><td>N</td><td>(5)</td></tr>
<tr><td>Mark the statement that is too broad</td><td>. . . . .</td><td>B</td><td>(5)</td></tr>
</table>

a. A quaking aspen has to make lots of seeds to get one successful sapling.

b. The seeds of quaking aspen have parachutes to help them float in the wind.

c. Quaking aspen can survive in harsh conditions where other trees cannot.

d. Trees have to be tough in order to survive in some places with harsh conditions.

Total Comprehension Score
(Add your scores and enter the
total on the graph on page 103.)

Categories of Comprehension Questions

No. 1: Subject Matter	No. 4: Clarifying Devices
No. 2: Supporting Details	No. 5: Vocabulary in Context
No. 3: Conclusion	No. 6: Main Idea

19. Squid

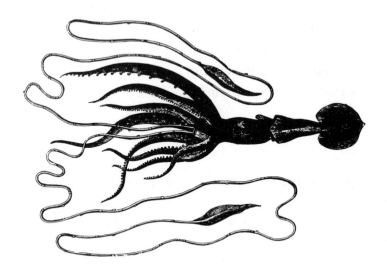

At a whaling station, some people were cutting up a sperm whale. They were getting ready to cook the pieces. But when they cut the stomach, a strange thing happened. A huge white body fell to the floor. It was a giant squid that had been swallowed whole!

The squid weighed 405 pounds (about 182.2 kilograms). It was 34 feet (about 10 meters) long from the tip of its tail to the tip of its long arms, or tentacles. Each eye was the size of a plate, over 7 inches (about 17.5 centimeters) across.

The biggest squid in the world live in the deep, dark, cold waters of the ocean. They have never been seen alive by people. They are so large that most fishing lines and nets can't hold them.

But scientists have learned a great deal about giant squid by studying parts of them found in whales' stomachs. They think that the largest squid may be as much as sixty feet (about 18.3 meters) long. They may weigh up to a ton (907.2 kilograms). They must be the largest *invertebrates* (animals with no backbones) in the world.

Most kinds of squid are smaller in size. They range from just a few inches (several centimeters) to forty feet (about 12.2 meters) in length.

Squid are sea mollusks. Clams, snails, and slugs are also in this species. But the squids have no outer shell. Buried in their flesh is a horny plate. Their closest kin is the octopus, which also has no outer shell.

Squid swim by squirting water from their body tube. They catch fish with their ten long arms, which are covered with sucking disks. They have webs between their tentacles which help them catch fish. All squid tear their food into bits with strong jaws like beaks.

	Possible Score	Your Score

1. What would be another good title for this passage?

   ☐ a. Giants of the Deep
   ☐ b. Jet Propulsion in the Squid
   ☐ c. Use Squid as Your Bait
   ☐ d. Tentacles of a Squid

   (15)   ◯

2. Squid are

   ☐ a. reptiles.
   ☐ b. sea mollusks.
   ☐ c. mammals.
   ☐ d. amphibians.

   (15)   ◯

3. Large squid have not been seen by people because

   ☐ a. they are shy and soon disappear from sight.
   ☐ b. they are very good at hiding.
   ☐ c. they live in very deep water.
   ☐ d. they are too dangerous to study.

   (15)   ◯

4. Most fishing lines and nets are made to hold

   ☐ a. very small fish.
   ☐ b. extra large fish.
   ☐ c. only shellfish.
   ☐ d. average-sized fish.

   (15)   ◯

5. A sucking disk is

   ☐ a. round.
   ☐ b. square.
   ☐ c. rectangular.
   ☐ d. triangular.

   (15)   ◯

6. Main Idea

	Answer	Score
Mark the main idea	M	(10)
Mark the statement that is a detail	D	(5)
Mark the statement that is too narrow	N	(5)
Mark the statement that is too broad	B	(5)

a. The sea contains many strange creatures.

b. Squid are unusual sea mollusks which vary greatly in size.

c. The giant squid may be the biggest of all animals without backbones.

d. The giant squid had eyes over seven inches (about 17.5 centimeters) across.

Total Comprehension Score
(Add your scores and enter the total on the graph on page 103.)

Categories of Comprehension Questions

No. 1: Subject Matter	No. 4: Clarifying Devices
No. 2: Supporting Details	No. 5: Vocabulary in Context
No. 3: Conclusion	No. 6: Main Idea

20. Traveling Seeds

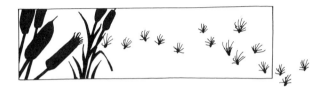

Most seeds that travel go by air. When you blow off a dandelion's soft white head, you are doing just what the wind does. You are spreading seeds. Dandelion and milkweed seeds have silky parachutes that help float them in the air. Cottonwood seeds have fine hairs that help them fly through the air.

Maple, elm and some pine seeds are like helicopters. They have wings that whirl in the wind. They go far from the parent trees.

There are seeds which are small and light. They need no parachutes, hairs or wings to help them fly. Airplanes have been used to collect grass seeds high up in the air! Orchid seeds are as fine as dust. Just one ripe orchid pod holds millions. If you breathe on them gently, they billow up like a cloud. The wind can blow tiny seeds like these for a few hundred miles or kilometers.

Other seeds use the wind to travel along the ground. Some seeds fall after the first snow. The wind then sends them sliding over the frozen ground. When the snow melts, they may sink down to the earth and start to grow.

Some seeds roll across the ground. Have you ever seen big, brown tumbleweeds blowing across a desert or prairie? When these bushes are full of ripe seeds, they dry out, and the roots <u>shrivel</u> up. Then the first wind to come along uproots the plant. It rolls along the ground, scattering seeds as it goes.

A few plants snap, crackle and pop. Tap the touch-me-not's seed pod, and it explodes with a *snap!* The pod is made of five little strips. These strips grow tighter and tighter over the seeds inside. When ripe, the strips spring apart at the slightest touch. They hit the seeds and flip them in all directions. The seed pod of the wild geranium is spring-loaded, too. But its seeds are on the springs. When the springs snap, they throw out the seeds the way you throw a baseball.

If you pinch a watermelon seed between your thumb and finger, it slips and pops away. This is how violet and witch hazel plants scatter their seeds. The sides of the seed pods open at one end. The pods squeeze harder and harder on the seeds inside. Pinch, POP!

Some seeds hitchhike. You might see your dog bite at a sticker in his fur. The sticker has hooks or claws which the seed uses to hitch a ride. Cockleburs, burdocks and stick-tights all travel like this. They are bitten, brushed or bumped off somewhere along the way. Then the seeds start a new pesky plant.

You help seeds travel, too. You can pop a touch-me-not, or cockleburs might stick to your socks. And where did you toss last summer's watermelon seeds?

?

	Possible Score	Your Score

1. This passage tell us

   ☐ a. why plants produce seeds.
   ☐ b. how seeds scatter.
   ☐ c. about edible seeds.
   ☐ d. what seeds need in order to grow.

   Possible Score (15) **Your Score** ○

2. Grass seeds have been found

   ☐ a. below the earth's surface.
   ☐ b. frozen in the Arctic wastelands.
   ☐ c. on the ocean floor.
   ☐ d. high in the air.

   (15) ○

3. In order to sprout, seeds usually

   ☐ a. move away from the parent plant.
   ☐ b. have to be big and heavy.
   ☐ c. need to be fertilized.
   ☐ d. become very cold and eventually pop.

   (15) ○

4. Maple, elm and pine seeds can be compared to helicopters because

   ☐ a. they do not glide when they fly.
   ☐ b. they can't stay in the air very long.
   ☐ c. they don't have parachutes.
   ☐ d. they have wings that whirl.

   (15) ○

5. A good synonym for shrivel is

   ☐ a. uproot.
   ☐ b. shrink.
   ☐ c. pop.
   ☐ d. swell.

   (15) ○

82

6. Main Idea

	Answer	Score
Mark the main idea	M	(10)
Mark the statement that is a detail	D	(5)
Mark the statement that is too narrow	N	(5)
Mark the statement that is too broad	B	(5)

a. Airplanes can collect grass seeds.

b. The wind blows some seeds hundred of miles or kilometers.

c. Seeds travel in several different ways.

d. Plants can start growing far from their parent plant.

Total Comprehension Score
(Add your scores and enter the total on the graph on page 103.)

Categories of Comprehension Questions

No. 1: Subject Matter	No. 4: Clarifying Devices
No. 2: Supporting Details	No. 5: Vocabulary in Context
No. 3: Conclusion	No. 6: Main Idea

21. Lizards and Their Habits

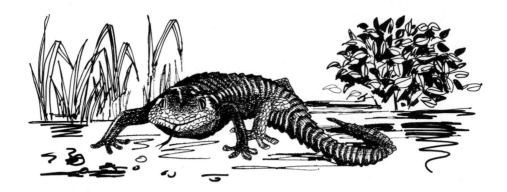

Lizards are reptiles like turtles and snakes. All reptiles are cold-blooded and have scales.

Unlike snakes, most lizards have four legs. Their feet have five toes. A few do have two legs and some have no legs at all! Most lizards have some sort of outside ear. Snakes do not. Most lizards can close their eyes. Snakes cannot.

Most lizards feed on insects, worms and other small creatures. All lizards munch on plants now and then. Some eat only plants.

The biggest lizard of all is called the *Komodo*. This one looks like a dragon from the past. It is found only on a few small islands in the South Seas. It can grow to be ten or twelve feet (about 3.1 or 3.7 meters) long. It can weigh as much as 300 pounds (about 136.1 kilograms)!

Once in a while it may bite a water buffalo or even a person. The victim will not die right there. But the liquid in the Komodo's mouth seems to have something in it that causes infection. The victim soon gets sick and dies.

Just two lizards are venomous. One of these lizards is the *gila* (HEE la) *monster* that lives in the deserts of our country. The other is a close cousin, the *beaded lizard* of Mexico.

At the far end of the lizard line are tiny ones just two inches (about 5.1 centimeters) long. They may weigh about an ounce (28.3 grams) or less. Between the huge and the tiny, lizards come in just about any size you would like to see.

Most lizards walk on all fours. Some move slowly. Others jump and dart about with great speed. Nothing seems to stop a lizard from getting where it wants to go. In tropical homes geckos go up walls and across ceilings with no trouble at all. They are welcome house guests because of the large number of insects which they catch and eat.

	Possible Score	Your Score

1. Lizards are

    ☐ a. snakes.
    ☐ b. reptiles.
    ☐ c. turtles.
    ☐ d. crocodiles.   (15)   ◯

2. All reptiles

    ☐ a. have 4 legs.
    ☐ b. are cold-blooded.
    ☐ c. are poisonous.
    ☐ d. cause infection.   (15)   ◯

3. The victim of the Komodo

    ☐ a. may suffer from rabies.
    ☐ b. does not die.
    ☐ c. dies immediately.
    ☐ d. dies from infection.   (15)   ◯

4. The last paragraph talks about

    ☐ a. favorite hiding places of reptiles.
    ☐ b. snake pets.
    ☐ c. lizards on the move.
    ☐ d. different sizes of reptiles.   (15)   ◯

5. A venomous lizard is

    ☐ a. poisonous.
    ☐ b. an amphibian.
    ☐ c. harmless.
    ☐ d. helpful.   (15)   ◯

6. Main Idea

	Answer	Score
Mark the main idea	M	(10)
Mark the statement that is a detail	D	(5)
Mark the statement that is too narrow	N	(5)
Mark the statement that is too broad	B	(5)

a. The reptile species contains creatures of wide variety.

b. Lizards vary in size, features and living habits.

c. Some lizards move slowly; some jump and dart about quickly.

d. A Komodo dragon is 10–12 feet (about 3.1–3.7 meters) long and can weigh 300 pounds (about 136.1 kilograms).

Total Comprehension Score
(Add your scores and enter the total on the graph on page 103.)

Categories of Comprehension Questions

No. 1: Subject Matter   No. 4: Clarifying Devices

No. 2: Supporting Details   No. 5: Vocabulary in Context

No. 3: Conclusion   No. 6: Main Idea

22. Home Sweet Home

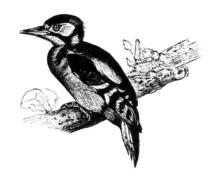

High in an old, dead tree, woodpeckers are working hard. They are trying to hollow out their nest. Then they line it with wood chips. The female lays a clutch of three to five eggs. Once the young hatch, the mother and father are kept busy. They search for food to feed their hungry newborns. Carpenter ants are one of their favorite foods. But they can eat other insects. They also eat wild fruit and berries. The parents take turns caring for the young, just as they did when making the nest. They both sat on the eggs to keep them warm.

Each day you return to the spot where you saw this ever-disappearing bird. Wait patiently for it to show itself again. One day you are rewarded. The woodpecker comes to search for food near your hiding place. You soon see how easily it tears bark from a dead pine. In about fifteen minutes it has peeled almost ten feet (about 3.1 meters) of bark off the tree in its hurried search for food.

Darting swiftly in and out, its long tongue searches for its target. The sticky coating on its tongue helps hold the insects captive until they are swallowed. Long toes with sharp, curved claws hold it safely on the branch.

All too soon it has finished its work. It flies off to take care of its hungry nestlings. Scramble to your feet. You can try to follow it to the nest. But the dense growth underfoot slows you down. Then it is gone. In the distance you can hear its loud, rasping "kuk-kuk" as it heads towards home.

?

	Possible Score	Your Score

1. This passage is about

   ☐ a. bats.
   ☐ b. a bird.
   ☐ c. raccoons.
   ☐ d. flying squirrels.

   (15)   ○

2. The female woodpecker lays

   ☐ a. 1 egg.
   ☐ b. 3–5 eggs.
   ☐ c. 7–10 eggs.
   ☐ d. 12 eggs.

   (15)   ○

3. We can see that young woodpeckers are cared for by

   ☐ a. both parents.
   ☐ b. the female only.
   ☐ c. the male only.
   ☐ d. neither parent.

   (15)   ○

4. The woodpecker in this story is looking for

   ☐ a. a nest.
   ☐ b. water.
   ☐ c. a mate.
   ☐ d. food.

   (15)   ○

5. A dense growth is

   ☐ a. thick.
   ☐ b. diseased.
   ☐ c. hollow.
   ☐ d. weak.

   (15)   ○

6. Main Idea

	Answer	Score
Mark the main idea	M	(10)
Mark the statement that is a detail	D	(5)
Mark the statement that is too narrow	N	(5)
Mark the statement that is too broad	B	(5)

a. Woodpeckers care for their young by hollowing out a nest and capturing insects for food.

b. Birds take good care of their young.

c. Woodpeckers build their nests inside old trees.

d. Woodpeckers have sticky coatings on their tongues to hold insects captive until they can be swallowed.

Total Comprehension Score
(Add your scores and enter the total on the graph on page 103.)

Categories of Comprehension Questions

No. 1: Subject Matter	No. 4: Clarifying Devices
No. 2: Supporting Details	No. 5: Vocabulary in Context
No. 3: Conclusion	No. 6: Main Idea

23. Time To Awaken

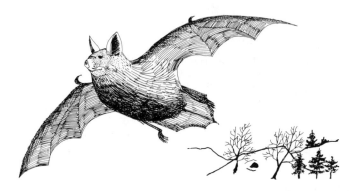

Long winter sleep, *hibernation,* ends quickly for some creatures, slowly for others. In the spring, the days grow long. The sun warms the soil. The eggs of the female grasshopper start to hatch. Out of the earth crawls a tiny creature. It seems to be all eyes and legs. In her life of just a few months this young grasshopper sheds her skin many times as she grows. She will be cursed by the farmer for the crops she eats. She will be caught by the farmer's child to make her "spit tobacco juice."

Come late summer, this grasshopper will listen <u>enthralled</u> to the "music" of a male who rubs his hind legs somewhere in the field. She will search him out. At last she finds the mate that can fertilize the eggs she carries in her body. Then, with the threat of the first frosts, she, too, will end her stay on earth by placing those eggs safely in the ground. In this way she provides for a new generation of her kind.

In his cave, the small brown bat has been lucky. The cave's temperature has been steady. If the cave had dropped below 30° Fahrenheit (-1.1° Celsius), the bat would have frozen. If it had risen above 40° Fahrenheit (4.4° Celsius) his body would have soon used up his stored fat. He would then have starved to death. Once in the winter the bat woke up enough to mate with a female nearby. He flew out of the cave for a few sips of water. Then once more he entered his state of sleep.

Now that the spring has come, the bat slowly stirs. He becomes active and hungry. Nearby, in a special section of the cave, the female gives birth. Hanging upside down, the female drops her young. She catches them in a pouch stretched on her wings made of the same membrane. In three weeks the young are ready to leave the cave in search of their own food. By August a young bat eats just as much as it can. It is storing fat for its long sleep. A young bat can double its weight in four to six weeks. Then, the cold descends across the forest and hills. The bat may seek the cave where it was born. There it passes into the long winter sleep that looks like death.

	Possible Score	Your Score

1. This passage focuses on the hibernation of

   ☐ a. the grasshopper and bat.
   ☐ b. the frog and bear.
   ☐ c. carp.
   ☐ d. reptiles.

   (15)   ○

2. If the temperature drops below 30° Fahrenheit (-1.1° Celsius), the brown bat will

   ☐ a. begin to hibernate.
   ☐ b. freeze to death.
   ☐ c. use up stored fat.
   ☐ d. become active.

   (15)   ○

3. Hibernation takes place

   ☐ a. during the winter.
   ☐ b. only on very cold days.
   ☐ c. during the mating season.
   ☐ d. during the spring and summer.

   (15)   ○

4. When a grasshopper "ends her stay on earth," she

   ☐ a. hibernates.
   ☐ b. dies.
   ☐ c. mates.
   ☐ d. finds a nest.

   (15)   ○

5. Another word for enthralled is

   ☐ a. bored.
   ☐ b. alarmed.
   ☐ c. fascinated.
   ☐ d. uninterested.

   (15)   ○

6. Main Idea

	Answer	Score
Mark the main idea	M	⑩
Mark the statement that is a detail	D	⑤
Mark the statement that is too narrow	N	⑤
Mark the statement that is too broad	B	⑤

a. Grasshopper eggs and adult bats hibernate all winter and become active in spring.

b. Many living creatures change their rates of activity in order to survive.

c. Grasshopper eggs stay quietly underground all winter before hatching.

d. A young bat can double its weight in four to six weeks.

Total Comprehension Score
(Add your scores and enter the total on the graph on page 103.)

Categories of Comprehension Questions

No. 1: Subject Matter	No. 4: Clarifying Devices
No. 2: Supporting Details	No. 5: Vocabulary in Context
No. 3: Conclusion	No. 6: Main Idea

24. Survival of the Fitter Nestling

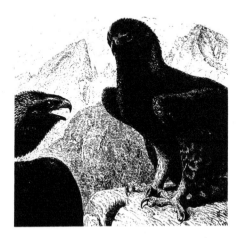

The two golden eaglets were less than a week old. They were almost helpless balls of white fluff. They barely had strength to raise their heads to be fed. The male eagle would bring fresh-killed meat. The female would tear it into bits to feed her young.

The male would also help repair the nest. He made four flights over the nest. He dropped leafy branches each time. Then he landed with a stick in his beak and passed it to the female. She pushed it into the nest. This kind of nest-building and repair goes on through the spring and summer until the eagles leave the aerie (AIR ee).

By the second week, one eaglet showed signs of dominating, or taking over, the nest and food. On my third visit, the weaker eaglet was gone from the nest. It may have starved.

By my fourth visit, the one eaglet left now had a black fringe on its wings and tail. It was growing fast. Food was always in the nest. The food was made up mostly of rabbits. I also saw the male bring one young badger and one bird. But the eaglet was not big enough to get a large share of the kill until it was close to a month old.

By the end of the sixth week, the young golden eagle had grown most of its feathers. A week later its <u>plumage</u> was starting to lighten. It soon showed more brown than black. I liked to watch the eaglet grow. But I couldn't help but think how only the strong survive in the animal world.

	Possible Score	Your Score

1. This passage talks mainly about

   ☐ a. the male eagle.
   ☐ b. young eagles.
   ☐ c. how eagles mate.   **15**   ◯
   ☐ d. the food of the eagle.

2. An eagle's nest is called an

   ☐ a. aerie.
   ☐ b. extension.
   ☐ c. arch.   **15**   ◯
   ☐ d. interval.

3. We can guess that the weak eagle died because

   ☐ a. the stronger eagle took all the food.
   ☐ b. it fell from the nest.
   ☐ c. the parents killed it.   **15**   ◯
   ☐ d. it froze to death.

4. In the last sentence, the writer sounds

   ☐ a. happy.
   ☐ b. excited.
   ☐ c. carefree.   **15**   ◯
   ☐ d. serious.

5. An eagle's <u>plumage</u> is its

   ☐ a. beak.
   ☐ b. claws.
   ☐ c. feathers.   **15**   ◯
   ☐ d. eyes.

6. Main Idea

	Answer	Score
Mark the main idea	M	(10)
Mark the statement that is a detail	D	(5)
Mark the statement that is too narrow	N	(5)
Mark the statement that is too broad	B	(5)

a. The weaker eaglet may have starved.

b. The male eagle helped feed the young.

c. Nature is not merciful to the weak.

d. Of the two eaglets, only the stronger survived.

Total Comprehension Score
(Add your scores and enter the
total on the graph on page 103.)

Categories of Comprehension Questions

No. 1: Subject Matter	No. 4: Clarifying Devices
No. 2: Supporting Details	No. 5: Vocabulary in Context
No. 3: Conclusion	No. 6: Main Idea

25. Buying Old, Old Coins

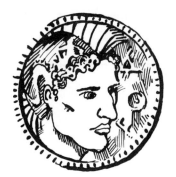 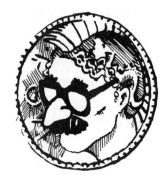

Many people want to buy old, old coins. But, before you part with your good money, watch out! You may be buying a coin that is really a fake.

Experts tell us that the making of fake coins goes back 2,000 years. In the old days, those who faked coins were punished with death. But now the making and selling of fake coins is a legal business.

Some of the fake coins are made so well that they are listed in coin books. And these coins are sought after by collectors. They will pay a high price for them.

It is one thing to buy a fake coin when it is sold as a fake. But it is another thing to buy a fake coin when it is sold as the real thing. The best advice is always buy from a reputable dealer. The dealer will take back a coin if it should prove to be a fake one.

But this advice is hard to follow if you visit other countries yourself. You might be tempted to buy coins "from the soil" rather than from a dealer. And many of these fake coins do come right from the soil. The fake coins are buried in secret. Then they are dug up in front of witnesses. The dealers themselves can be fooled by this.

Another trick is for someone who sells postcards to have one fake coin. It is a copy of a rare coin and is placed among some real but common coins. The visitor sees the real coins. The visitor thinks then that the rare coin is real too. When this happens, the visitor has been tricked. So, if you decide to buy old coins, be careful!

?

	Possible Score	Your Score

1. This passage is mainly about

   ☐ a. today's coins.
   ☐ b. how old coins were made.
   ☐ c. fake coins.
   ☐ d. coin collectors.

   (15) ○

2. This passage tells of coins

   ☐ a. in your country.
   ☐ b. in other countries.
   ☐ c. on the ocean floor.
   ☐ d. found in caves.

   (15) ○

3. People who are tricked into buying fake coins are most often

   ☐ a. coin collectors.
   ☐ b. people who stay at home.
   ☐ c. antique dealers.
   ☐ d. visitors to another country.

   (15) ○

4. The last sentence is trying

   ☐ a. to warn the reader.
   ☐ b. to be humorous.
   ☐ c. to compare coins.
   ☐ d. to explain coin collecting.

   (15) ○

5. A reputable dealer is one who is

   ☐ a. small.
   ☐ b. a city worker.
   ☐ c. friendly.
   ☐ d. trustworthy.

   (15) ○

6. Main Idea

	Answer	Score
Mark the main idea	M	(10)
Mark the statement that is a detail	D	(5)
Mark the statement that is too narrow	N	(5)
Mark the statement that is too broad	B	(5)

a. Making fake coins goes back 2,000 years.

b. There are many ways people can be tricked into buying fake coins.

c. Some coin dealers pretend they have dug up fake coins from the soil.

d. Things may not be what they appear to be.

Total Comprehension Score
(Add your scores and enter the
total on the graph on page 103.)

Categories of Comprehension Questions

No. 1: Subject Matter	No. 4: Clarifying Devices
No. 2: Supporting Details	No. 5: Vocabulary in Context
No. 3: Conclusion	No. 6: Main Idea

Acknowledgments

The passages appearing in this book have been reprinted with the kind permission of the following publications and publishers to whom the author is indebted:

Aramco World Magazine, published by The Arabian American Oil Company, New York, New York.

The Communicator, published by the New York State Outdoor Education Association, Syracuse, New York.

The Conservationist, published by the New York State Conservation Department, Albany, New York.

A Cornell Science Leaflet, published by the New York State College of Agriculture and Life Sciences, a unit of the State University, at Cornell University, Ithaca, New York.

Food, The Yearbook of Agriculture, published by the United States Department of Agriculture, Washington, D.C.

Handbook of Nature-Study, published by Comstock Publishing Company, Ithaca, New York.

Kansas Fish & Game, published by the Kansas Forestry, Fish and Game Commission, Pratt, Kansas.

National Wildlife, published by The National Wildlife Federation, Washington, D.C.

Outdoor Oklahoma, published by the Oklahoma Department of Wildlife Conservation, Oklahoma City, Oklahoma.

Pennsylvania Game News, published by the Pennsylvania Game Commission, Harrisburg, Pennsylvania.

Ranger Rick's Nature Magazine, published by The National Wildlife Federation, Washington, D.C.

The Tennessee Conservationist, published by the Tennessee Department of Conservation and the Tennessee Game and Fish Commission.

Answer Key: Book 2

Passage 1:	1.a	2.d	3.a	4.c	5.c	6a.**M**	6b.**N**	6c.**B**	6d.**D**
Passage 2:	1.c	2.a	3.d	4.c	5.d	6a.**N**	6b.**B**	6c.**D**	6d.**M**
Passage 3:	1.c	2.a	3.d	4.d	5.c	6a.**M**	6b.**D**	6c.**B**	6d.**N**
Passage 4:	1.b	2.a	3.d	4.c	5.a	6a.**D**	6b.**N**	6c.**B**	6d.**M**
Passage 5:	1.b	2.b	3.a	4.b	5.d	6a.**D**	6b.**M**	6c.**B**	6d.**N**
Passage 6:	1.d	2.a	3.a	4.b	5.d	6a.**N**	6b.**M**	6c.**D**	6d.**B**
Passage 7:	1.c	2.b	3.d	4.a	5.b	6a.**B**	6b.**D**	6c.**M**	6d.**N**
Passage 8:	1.c	2.d	3.b	4.b	5.c	6a.**B**	6b.**D**	6c.**M**	6d.**N**
Passage 9:	1.b	2.d	3.b	4.d	5.a	6a.**D**	6b.**M**	6c.**B**	6d.**N**
Passage 10:	1.d	2.b	3.d	4.c	5.a	6a.**B**	6b.**D**	6c.**M**	6d.**N**
Passage 11:	1.d	2.b	3.a	4.c	5.d	6a.**B**	6b.**D**	6c.**N**	6d.**M**
Passage 12:	1.c	2.b	3.b	4.a	5.c	6a.**B**	6b.**M**	6c.**D**	6d.**N**
Passage 13:	1.b	2.d	3.a	4.d	5.b	6a.**N**	6b.**M**	6c.**B**	6d.**D**

Passage 14:	1.**a**	2.**b**	3.**b**	4.**c**	5.**a**	6a.**N**	6b.**B**	6c.**D**	6d.**M**
Passage 15:	1.**c**	2.**d**	3.**a**	4.**d**	5.**a**	6a.**B**	6b.**N**	6c.**D**	6d.**M**
Passage 16:	1.**c**	2.**b**	3.**a**	4.**d**	5.**b**	6a.**M**	6b.**D**	6c.**B**	6d.**N**
Passage 17:	1.**b**	2.**d**	3.**b**	4.**a**	5.**d**	6a.**N**	6b.**B**	6c.**M**	6d.**D**
Passage 18:	1.**c**	2.**d**	3.**b**	4.**c**	5.**c**	6a.**N**	6b.**D**	6c.**M**	6d.**B**
Passage 19:	1.**a**	2.**b**	3.**c**	4.**d**	5.**a**	6a.**B**	6b.**M**	6c.**N**	6d.**D**
Passage 20:	1.**b**	2.**d**	3.**a**	4.**d**	5.**b**	6a.**D**	6b.**N**	6c.**M**	6d.**B**
Passage 21:	1.**b**	2.**b**	3.**d**	4.**c**	5.**a**	6a.**B**	6b.**M**	6c.**N**	6d.**D**
Passage 22:	1.**b**	2.**b**	3.**a**	4.**d**	5.**a**	6a.**M**	6b.**B**	6c.**N**	6d.**D**
Passage 23:	1.**a**	2.**b**	3.**a**	4.**b**	5.**c**	6a.**M**	6b.**B**	6c.**N**	6d.**D**
Passage 24:	1.**b**	2.**a**	3.**a**	4.**d**	5.**c**	6a.**N**	6b.**D**	6c.**B**	6d.**M**
Passage 25:	1.**c**	2.**b**	3.**d**	4.**a**	5.**d**	6a.**D**	6b.**M**	6c.**N**	6d.**B**

Diagnostic Chart (For Student Correction)

Directions: Write your final answers in the *upper* part of the passage block. Then correct your answers using the Answer Key on pages 100 and 101. If your answer is correct, do not make any more marks in the block. If your answer is incorrect, write the letter of the correct answer in the *lower* part of the block.

Reading Passage

Categories of Comprehension Skills	1	2	3	4	5	6	7	8	9	10	11	12	13	14	15	16	17	18	19	20	21	22	23	24	25
1. Subject Matter																									
2. Supporting Details																									
3. Conclusion																									
4. Clarifying Devices																									
5. Vocabulary in Context																									
6. Main Idea — Main Idea																									
Detail																									
Too Narrow																									
Too Broad																									

Progress Graph

Directions: Write your Total Comprehension Score in the box under the number for each passage. Then put an *x* along the line above each box to show your Total Comprehension Score for that passage. Then make a graph of your progress. Draw a line to connect the *x*'s.

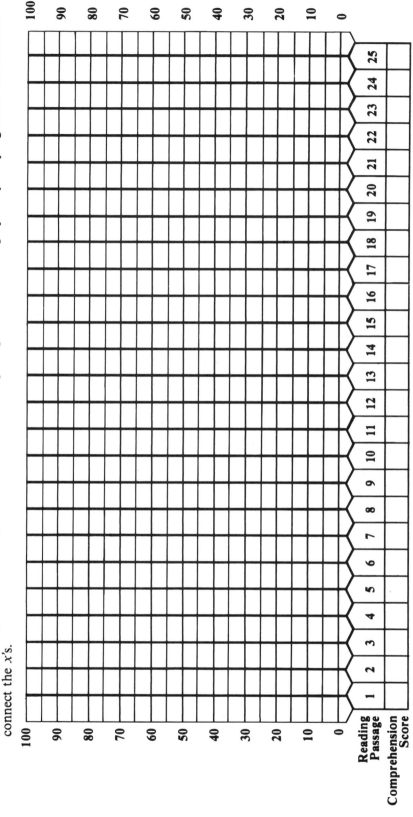

Reading Passage	1	2	3	4	5	6	7	8	9	10	11	12	13	14	15	16	17	18	19	20	21	22	23	24	25
Comprehension Score																									

Classroom
Management
System

Essential Skills Series

Classroom Management System
(For Teacher Correction)

To the Teacher

The Classroom Management System provides an easy and effective way to individualize instruction. It can be used by reading specialists as well as by regular classroom teachers. The management system is designed to be equally effective when used with a single student, a small group, or a full-size class.

The Classroom Management System provides ongoing assessment of student work for both you and your student. It shows not only the amount of work completed, but also the quality of the work.

It serves as a diagnostic tool by revealing patterns of errors at a glance. For example, if a student has difficulty identifying subject matter (question #1 in each set of questions throughout the *Essential Skills Series*), a pattern of errors will appear in the Subject Matter column of the Classroom Management System Record Sheet. This will enable you to focus on the specific skills needs of each student.

The Classroom Management System Record Sheet is on pages 108-109. Both pages may be duplicated and stapled together.

How to Use the Classroom Management System Record Sheet

Step 1: Have the student answer the questions for each *Essential Skills* passage under the appropriate question heading.

Passage	① Subject Matter	② Supporting Details	③ Conclusion	④ Clarifying Devices	⑤ Vocabulary in Context	⑥ Main Idea				Number Correct	Errors Corrected
						a	b	c	d		
1	d	c	a	b	d			N D B M			

Step 2: Circle any incorrect answers and fill in the total number correct.

1	d	c	a	b	d			N D B M	6

Step 3: Have the student correct his or her incorrect answers.

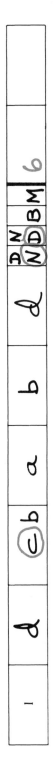

Step 4: Give assistance as needed and, if necessary, correct the student's adjusted answers.

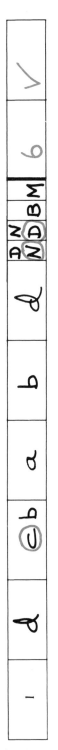

Step 5: Have the student go on to the next passage.

Step 6: Repeat Steps 1-4. If the class is large, it may be necessary to have students complete two or three passages before you correct them. This will slow the "traffic" at your desk.

Note: It is important for students to analyze and, to the extent possible, correct their own errors (Step 3).

Essential Skills Series

Classroom Management System Record Sheet
(For Teacher Correction)

Name _____

Teacher _____

Date _____

Book Number _____

To the Student: Write your answers in the spaces provided. (See the Example below.) Your teacher will circle any incorrect answers. Then go back over the questions and correct your mistakes.

Passage	① Subject Matter	② Supporting Details	③ Conclusion	④ Clarifying Devices	⑤ Vocabulary in Context	⑥ Main Idea a	b	c	d	Number Correct	Errors Corrected
Example	c	ⓑ a	d	a	c	a	ⓝⓓⓜ		ⓑ		
1											
2											
3											
4											
5											
6											
7											
8											
9											
10											

	1	2	3	4	5	6		
11								
12								
13								
14								
15								
16								
17								
18								
19								
20								
21								
22								
23								
24								
25								

This record sheet may be duplicated for classroom use by teachers.
From *Essential Skills Series* by Walter Pauk, copyright © 1982 by Jamestown Publishers. Classroom Management System by Thomas F. Kelly, Ph.D.